ADHD and Success at Work

Heiner Lachenmeier

ADHD and Success at Work

How to turn supposed shortcomings into strengths

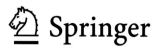 Springer

Heiner Lachenmeier
Affoltern am Albis, Switzerland

Translated by
Mrs. Julia Thornton

ISBN 978-3-031-13436-4   ISBN 978-3-031-13437-1   (eBook)
https://doi.org/10.1007/978-3-031-13437-1

Translation from the German language edition: "Mit ADHS erfolgreich im Beruf" by Heiner Lachenmeier,
© © 2020 Springer Nature Switzerland AG. Part of Springer Nature 2021. Published by SpringerNature.
All Rights Reserved.

This Springer imprint is published by the registered company Springer Nature Switzerland AG
The registered company address is: Gewerbestrasse 11, 6330 Cham, Switzerland

For Anna, Nara and Gabriela

Preface for the English Edition

In the introduction to the original German edition, I wrote that in order to deal with ADHD successfully, we need comprehensible models of how it functions. I was astonished to receive many letters and emails from ADHDers throughout Switzerland, Germany and Austria, who told me that for the first time they understood why they felt and behaved the way they did. A 30-year-old engineer from Munich described that it was almost embarrassing when he read about typical ADHD problems in puberty that so closely resembled his own experience; it was as if he himself had served as the template for them. He emphasised "almost" because the relief of understanding at last how he came to find himself with these kinds of problems and of learning to master them better than before was overwhelming. But most of the feedback was of course related to workplace issues and the relief of finally understanding how the functionality of ADHD was a contributing factor. On top of that even getting tips on how on earth to overcome them at last.

A growing number of requests about an English edition, both from ADHDers and professionals, soon made it clear to me that this had to be done. It was a stroke of luck to find Mrs Julia Thornton, a British-born musician and translator living in Germany. She not only translated the book in a short space of time but proved to show a deep understanding of the text and was able to communicate the meaning as well as its tone in her translation. A big thank you!

Last but not least I thank my family, first and foremost my partner Gabriela Frischknecht who supports me with her love and her professionalism, and my children Anna and Nara, who make me proud to be their father.

Affoltern am Albis/Scuol, Switzerland   Heiner Lachenmeier
July 2022

Preface

This book is primarily aimed at people with ADHD who want to get along better in their working lives. It can also be a helpful read for their superiors, subordinates, colleagues and for human resources (HR) staff. Relatives may find it useful, too. And not least, it is intended to give medical specialists practice-based tips for tangible, viable treatment options.

The text is illustrated, served up in small portions, highly subdivided for better readability, and clarified with easily understandable case studies. I have sectioned off interesting supplementary information under the heading "Encore" in grey highlighted boxes. If readers are in a hurry, they can skip these sections. To hold the readers' attention, I have written in a conversational tone. This is a common courtesy when writing a book for ADHDers. And I admit that this also made the many hours of writing it easier, because I could simply recount things.

I suspect that readers may consult individual chapters, if the corresponding issues apply to them, without reading the whole book. I have therefore repeated important content several times, meaning that the sections can always be understood, even if they are read in isolation.

The filter and control models of ADHD have been described in academic literature for many years. In this book, the relationship of these models to everyday tangible reality—to the experience of ADHDers—has been identified and presented in a new way. The differentiated conceptualisation of various characteristics of ADHD such as different learning curves, negative hyperfocus, emergency benefit, self-perception falsification, Mount Everest syndrome, etc. as well as the coping mechanisms and treatment recommendations derived from these characteristics are derived from my experience and practical research.

Some people have accused me of being too casual in referring to "ADHDers". Since I am an ADHDer too, I have allowed myself to use this nonchalant figure of speech. It is simply easier than the clumsy and somewhat debilitating term "person with ADHD".

In line with the conventions of Springer Publishing, to improve readability I have sometimes used the masculine pronouns "he", "him", "his" when referring to "people in a general sense" and would like to stress that I include all gender variations here.

I needed a great deal of support in writing this book and would particularly like to thank lic. phil. Gabriela Frischknecht, who kept me decisively on course, not only as a critic beyond compare in this field, but also as my life partner. I am also grateful to my two adult children, Anna and Nara, who taught me a great deal, with protestations and good humour. Thanks also go to Werner Fuchs, whose clear-sighted and sharp professionalism prevented me from losing my way in the world of publishing. What's more, he put me in touch with Emil Gut, a graphic designer who immediately understood what I wanted to visualise and how. Special thanks go to Katrin Lenhart and Christiane Beisel from Springer Publishing for all their patience and support.

And finally, I would like to thank the many people I have come to know as patients. I am very conscious of the fact that without their shared experiences, I would have acquired a great deal of knowledge, admittedly, but have been unable to truly understand anything.

Affoltern am Albis, Switzerland   Heiner Lachenmeier

Contents

About the Author

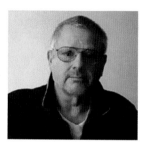

Heiner Lachenmeier Specialist in psychiatry & psychotherapy

Lachenmeier was first diagnosed with ADHD when he was middle-aged, although there were more than enough signs of it when he was a child. He climbed up every tree—and sometimes crashed down out of them. He also crashed out of one academic high school as the worst pupil in the class—and was top of the class in the next one.

He studied medicine at the University of Basle and did his doctorate at the University of Zurich. He trained as a specialist in psychiatry and psychotherapy. During the 1990s, he established and was director of the Swiss Training Institute for Analytical Short-term Psychotherapy (GIK). Lachenmeier's involvement in the policies of his profession includes membership of the executive board of the Swiss Society for Psychiatry and Psychotherapy (SGPP) and the Swiss Medical Association (FMH). In 2002 he brought the Swiss specialist psychiatric associations together into one collective umbrella organisation (FMPP) which he subsequently presided over.

Lachenmeier has focused on ADHD in adults for around 20 years. He focuses on researching how ADHD functions, its relevance to how ADHDers experience the condition, and implementing his observations in practice-based models to explain and treat ADHD. He coaches executives with ADHD as well as the managers of employees with ADHD. He undertakes a wide range of activities as a lecturer, supervisor and coach.

Heiner Lachenmeier is divorced and the father of two adult children. With his life partner lic. phil Gabriela Frischknecht, a specialist in psychotherapy, he runs a psychiatric-psychotherapeutic specialist practice near Zurich. Together they give seminars and courses on ADHD as well as ADHD and gestalt therapy.

Heiner Lachenmeier is an honorary member of the Aargau Society for Psychiatry and Psychotherapy and an honorary member of the Swiss self-help organisation adhs20plus; he is also a member of several professional associations such as the Swiss Society for ADHD (SFG ADHS), ADD-Forum Berlin and the World Federation of ADHD.

List of Case Studies

Introduction

As people, we need to be able to understand our world. This applies whether we are the so-called "little ones" or fully fledged adults. Understanding our world enables us to find and follow our path in it.

Understanding is much deeper than just knowledge. Knowledge is something you can learn off by heart. If I learn off by heart from a tour description that I need to turn right on a mountain bike tour at a specific coordinate, then I could actually have a fatal accident if I strictly followed this knowledge. Perhaps a piece of rock has slid down, a chasm in the path has been created and I will need to turn right earlier. Every sensible person would understand this when looking at the path and would not stubbornly follow the coordinates they have learned—although some of us, blindly following the "knowledge" of our satnavs, have ended up with our car in a field.

Today's psychiatric and psychological diagnoses system is much too strongly based on fragmented-statistic knowledge of a very limited number of possible symptoms. As a consequence, quite a few specialists do not seek, as a matter of course, to understand human existence and suffering. Neither in terms of fundamental human insight, nor in terms of understanding the individual person. They neglect to understand contexts, processes, interrelationships and developments (Andreasen 2007).

But the fact is that the more in-depth we understand something, the better we can deal with it. It's more likely that we will be able to find practical solutions if we have any difficulties. In the example quoted above, we naturally adapt our route to the changed circumstances. Without a fundamental understanding of the terrain, with the isolated knowledge of the route coordinates we would be stranded in front of the rockfall, unable to act, or we would stubbornly continue on the original route and fall down.

H. Lachenmeier, *ADHD and Success at Work*, https://doi.org/10.1007/978-3-031-13437-1_1

ADHD Means Being a Little Different in This World

Everyone needs an understanding of their environment and themselves. What if you belonged to a large group of people, although compared with the entire humanity, actually a small group of people, who function slightly differently than the average person? How much more important it would be for you to understand how you yourself tick? And how & where other people tick differently?

According to the current state of knowledge, around 5% of people have ADHD (Barkley 2017). I deliberately didn't write "…suffer from…". Not all of them suffer from having ADHD. And a whole lot of them suffer less from ADHD itself but much more from the fact that they do not understand it and therefore get repeatedly entangled in misunderstandings and conflicts.

We therefore need plausible models which enable us to understand ADHD. This is a prerequisite for being able to find our path in life with ADHD—particularly in our working lives—without unnecessary conflict. If we are able to understand this, even if only partly, we are often able to deal with most life situations in a sufficiently appropriate and flexible way. In short: with less trouble and more success.

At this point and for the first time, I would like to emphasis the term "sufficient". It's about a "sufficient" understanding and also "sufficient" implementation of tasks. Perfectionism can definitely be important in special situations and areas, but in everyday life, it's only rarely a good idea and sometimes even obstructive and can even create a total block.

It's about having clearly understandable, plausible models of ADHD.

A model is developed using various elements. In them, findings from fundamental research (above all neurobiology, genetics and pharmacology) as well as other insights from the fields of psychology and psychiatry are processed. However, the absolutely essential fundamental elements are the experiences reported by people with ADHD as well as the behavioural patterns and processes observed externally. A model should be able to bring the different elements into a logically plausible correlation.

In this way, a model serves as a kind of functional overview; the basis for understanding people with ADHD, including their emotional contexts.

This must be possible in a linguistically simple way, without excessive terminology such as synapse, prefrontal, striatum, limbic system, amygdala, locus coeruleus and so on. We need correct but generally understandable terms that are specific and useful.

For example, you can explain football simply: two teams with 11 players, one defined field, two goals, one ball, a few other basic rules—and you have to kick the round thing into the net. Everyone understands this—it's sufficient as a simple plausible basic model. The game can begin—it doesn't matter if this means you start to play yourself, or you want to watch from the side.

Of course, there are subtleties when it comes to the rules; there can even be a high degree of differentiation. But they do not help those who want to get to know the world of football to understand it further. It's better to do this by simply describing the emotions during a match and having the miserable experience of being kicked in the shins.

Naturally, these models and characteristics won't always be exactly the same as a person's individually experienced reality. Please regard them as a *preliminary* result from decades of practical research. Both the basic research and practical research will bring further insights and developments. And not least, the experiences, self-observations and reflections of people with ADHD will make up an essential element in improving the understanding of ADHD.

I hope that university research will increasingly take up the insights from practical research and patient experiences and with the funds available to it, and undertake research at least as actively as the sometimes banal/self-evident correlations à la "we have scientifically statistically proven that the more strongly pronounced ADHD is in the person affected, the more stress they have".

Verification or falsification of models and their importance in understanding and coping with ADHD, as well as their consequences for therapeutic approaches would be a much richer field for smart scientists.

Encore

To you, dear reader, I have one simple request: if you notice inconsistencies, have something to add, additional information, observations or ideas, then please contribute them. Whether it's as feedback to me, to the doctor treating you, in discussion with colleagues, via an ADHD chat or to another suitable place, generally in the spirit of an "open-source mentality".

You should assume that there is still plenty to be discovered, particularly by those affected themselves. Perhaps no-one else has realised yet, what you have noticed.

Back to ADHD and the world of work. The aim of this book is to help you understand ADHD better and enable you to release more of your potential.

References

Andreasen NC. DSM and the death of phenomenology in America: an example of unintended consequences. Schizophr Bull. 2007;33(1):108–12.
Barkley RA. Das grosse Handbuch für Erwachsene mit ADHS. Bern: Hogrefe; 2017.

One Person's ADHD Is Not the Same as Another's

2

2.1   ADHD Can Make Work More Difficult *and* Make It Easier

ADHD plays a role at work and in the world of work.

Sometimes positive; sometimes negative. The size of this role, and how exactly it has an effect depend on many other factors in the individual case. Below I will explain the functional pattern of ADHD in typical situations and deduce from this how you can minimise or even avoid damage.

Or even better: how you can realise the possible benefits of ADHD.

Case Study 1

From Loser to Achiever of the Year

Alfons was a young man, very sporty, usually cheerful and seemingly happy, but with an enormous amount of hidden self-doubt and insecurity. During his schooldays, he got into difficulties with fellow pupils and teaching staff owing to his impulsiveness. He didn't seem very interested in school, didn't get good results and was known more for his disruptive behaviour. After his compulsory schooling he did a trade apprenticeship as there weren't many other alternatives, simply because there was still a place free there. He just about got through his training, spent most of the time doing sport, drank too much alcohol and therefore had to give up his driving licence shortly after passing his driving test. After completing his apprenticeship, his trainer was glad to see the back of him.

H. Lachenmeier, *ADHD and Success at Work*, https://doi.org/10.1007/978-3-031-13437-1_2

At first glance, he seemed predestined to have a career as a loser. After the apprenticeship, Alfons found a job in a company for automatised building parts. He had absolutely no idea about this work, but shortly after starting the job he noticed that he was interested in it. Alfons read everything he could get his hands upon in order to understand the mechanical parts, the electronic control systems and the software behind it.

While he did this, he had to rush from building site to building site, and for months felt as if he didn't understand anything. He couldn't connect the theory he was reading about with his practical everyday work. He began to have more and more self-doubts. After about a year, he shyly asked his foreman why a particularly building component was constructed in one specific way, and not in a different way: it would be easier to install if a small change was made, and the component would probably last longer.

Nobody listened to his suggestion. "Just do your work", or "So you think you're an engineer, do you?" were phrases that he kept hearing. Despite this, Alfons set about making a prototype with a colleague who owned a lathe and a milling machine.

Then he went to the boss of the workshop, who was also an ADHDer—something which Alfons didn't realise at the time, however. The workshop boss recognised the advantages of Alfons' component immediately. Together they got in touch with the company owner and were able to start a test series.

The component proved to be a success. This small company went on to save several millions of francs per year because of it, and client satisfaction also improved. The "predestined loser" now works in the development division, although he is not yet 30 years old, and is rightly a member of the management. The company has expanded thanks to several of Alfons' innovations.

- As well as Alfons' ability to innovate, decisive factors for this company were that one of his superiors noticed his potential, the company managers deployed him unbureaucratically in a position where he functioned best and enabled him to undertake targeted further training.

  If Alfons had got no further than the reaction of the foreman, it would have been a great loss for the company

- For Alfons himself, a decisive factor was that in the years earlier he had learned how his ADHD functioned, meaning that he could minimise the disadvantages and maximise the advantages.

  This helped Alfons to deal better with the initial rejection of the foreman. He found a constructive route. Without knowing about how his ADHD functions, he would have reacted impulsively to the frustration, got drunk and regarded himself as a victim of the "stupid boss". As this kind of reaction is usually not a single occurrence, he would probably have been predestined for a career as a "loser".

2.2   "Unusual Management of Information and Functions"

If we consider ADHD from an exclusively symptom-based point of view, we get an incoherent range of possible symptoms, some of them catastrophic (APA 2015) and no perspective on any of the equally possible advantages.

This one-sided view of symptoms is unfair and disheartening to those persons affected. It doesn't help us in understanding ADHD either, leads to diverse misunderstandings and ultimately hampers constructive collaboration.

If we want to find ways of understanding ADHD, then it's worth taking a functional perspective with which we can understand ADHD phenomena as far as possible and learn to recognise their characteristics. We can then deduce several solution approaches (see below for concrete examples).

This starts already with the name of the condition:

In the term "attention deficit and hyperactivity disorder", the words "deficit" and "disorder" are emphasised. Two particularly conspicuous symptoms thereby receive too much importance and distract us from the essence of ADHD.

It would be more appropriate—and the entire breadth of possible positive and negative phenomena would be correctly covered—to speak of UMIF:

Unusual Management of Information and Functions

> because with ADHD, it's not just about recognising **symptoms.**
> Nor about the **functionality** of ADHD;
> rather, it's about their **SIGNIFICANCE**
> for the experiences, reactions and behaviour
> of the person affected,
> particularly their **emotional** significance.

In recent years it has been recognised that, contrary to earlier beliefs, ADHD and high-functioning autism can occur simultaneously and exhibit several overlaps (Philipsen 2013). From this point of view, too, a designation that takes the unusual management of information and functions into consideration seems to be a better idea than one that is unnecessarily pathologising.

Nevertheless, to avoid causing confusion, I will use the conventional term ADHD in this book, and I will not differentiate between ADHD and ADD for the same reason.

2.3   Personality

As well as the fundamental way that ADHD functions, and its severity, there are other individual factors that play a role. In brief: the ***personality*** and the path taken through life until now.

For example, a high level of intelligence can be used to establish a systematic sifting and weighting of information as a way of coping (see Sect. 3.3), with which an ADHDer can get a rapid overview of an excessive amount of information (see Sect. 3.1).

This functions above all when good intelligence is paired with a supporting and respectful upbringing—if the person therefore has optimal chances to develop a more or less good perception of their self-worth.

If a strong sense of self-doubt develops above all, then a high level of intelligence can also lead to a very great sense of insecurity—the higher the intelligence, the larger the association trees. This can rapidly lead to a kind of blockage in different areas of our lives, particularly in our professional lives.

A person's individual interests also play a major role. If these coincidentally happen to be important school subjects, then this ADHDer will usually be significantly less conspicuous in school than an ADHDer of the same intelligence, whose interests are painting and mountaineering. The possible influence on later consequences at work is obvious.

2.4   Environment

The *social environment* also plays an important role for everyone, but often a significantly larger one for ADHDers. The surfeit of information can create a kind of "fog", which makes it difficult to get an overall view of things, and which leads to more insecurity. It becomes even more important for ADHDers to have people and structures towards which they can orient themselves.

2.4.1   Focus on People

Comparison: all first year primary school pupils, with or without ADHD, are broadly dependent on having a clear and good relationship with their teacher in order to be able to concentrate and find their way in the big new world of school.

ADHDers are often very much more dependent on these kinds of positive relationships in order to unleash their potential at later stages of their career—during an apprenticeship, during higher education study, or throughout their whole lives. These relationships could be with a trainer, a manager or even an identity-giving community; through which there is an increased risk of a dependency developing.

This means that the luck of having a teacher or manager who fits can have a far greater influence on whether an ADHDer has a successful career or not.

2.4.2   Focus on Structures

Clear and constructive structures with a certain amount of freedom—a so-called appreciative discipline command, can be very beneficial. This is the complete opposite of rigid, inflexible derogatory discipline coercion.

This can concern structures within the family, the close social environment but also the respective dominant contemporary and political parameters. Structures play a major role in whether ADHDers can prove themselves occupationally.

Naturally the different ways that ADHD functions, the other individual factors and the environmental factors can all have mutually influenced each other and may continue to do so in the future.

References

American Psychiatric Association. Diagnostisches und Statistisches Manual Psychischer Störungen DSM-%. Bern: Hogrefe; 2015.

Philipsen A. Autismus-Spektrum-Störungen und Aufmerksamkeitsdefizit-Hyperaktivitätsstörung. In: Tebartz van Elst l (pub.). Das Asperger-Syndrom im Erwachsenenalter. Berlin: Medizinisch Wissenschaftliche Verlagsgesellschaft; 2013.

The Functional System of ADHD

It's Not That ADHDers Think Too Little: They Just Think Too Widely

ADHD is a genetic condition (Faraone 2004) with advantages and disadvantages.

Additional factors play a role in whether and how strongly ADHD causes problems in individuals and whether it qualifies as an illness.

> **Encore**
> The genetic condition ADHD is not an illness in itself but a normal variant seen in a percentage of the population. For example, being a man or being a woman is a normal variant. Nobody would come to the conclusion that just because specific diseases are seen in men and women (e.g. testicular cancer or cervical cancer), that being a man or a woman is in itself an illness.

Important: when I describe possible ADHD phenomena and symptoms in this book, then this does not mean every ADHDer necessarily exhibits all the manifestations of them. The fundamental mechanisms are the same; but the "configuration" is individual.

3.1 Information: Weighting and Filtering—The Filter Model

Information is less automatically weighted or filtered (Fig. 3.1):

- Information from outside (input)
- Information from your own storage system (memory)
- Linking information from these two sources (thinking, associating and feeling accordingly)

H. Lachenmeier, *ADHD and Success at Work*, https://doi.org/10.1007/978-3-031-13437-1_3

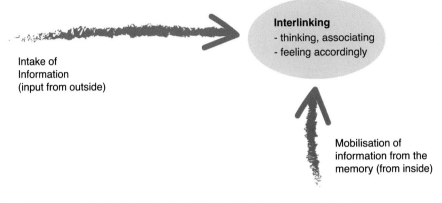

Intake of
Information
(input from outside)

Interlinking
- thinking, associating
- feeling accordingly

Mobilisation of
information from the
memory (from inside)

Fig. 3.1   ADHD basics: in these three places, information is less pre-filtered

In the case of ADHD, there is less dopamine and less noradrenaline available in these areas (Trott 1993). Dopamine dampens down less important information, whereas noradrenaline strengthens important information. This means that important information is emphasised in comparison to unimportant information (Stieglitz and Hofecker-Fallahpour 2007).

Dopamine and noradrenaline therefore have a kind of navigation function which is reduced if ADHD is present. Or put another way: ADHDers need to process more data.

This results in a difference in the perception and processing of information (Armstrong et al. 2001).

In brief, this means that non-ADHDers get a faster overview whereas ADHDers have a wider breadth of association. These are the basic forms of how non-ADHD and ADHD function, and represent the basis for understanding ADHD and non-ADHD. In illustrations 3.2 to 3.4, they are depicted together with their respective characteristic effects.

ADHDers therefore continually need to process more information than non-ADHDers. The way in which individuals deal with the surfeit of information differs greatly; it can be more or less effective but is on the whole very resourceful. The overcoming or dealing with the flood of data is described using the terms "coping" and "coping mechanisms" (read more about coping in Sect. 3.3).

The fundamental differences between ADHD and non-ADHD are concealed by the diverse coping mechanisms. **The depiction of the basic forms of ADHD and non-ADHD does not include any coping mechanisms** (Figs. 3.2 and 3.3).

This automatic pre-filtering makes it enormously easier for non-ADHDers to deal with the tasks of everyday life. This is extremely practical and highly efficient.

On the other hand, this automatic pre-filter has an effect similar to a "pre-censor" in non-ADHDers, although this is an extreme and not quite correct way of putting it. To put it more correctly: non-ADHDers are partly limited to the framework of

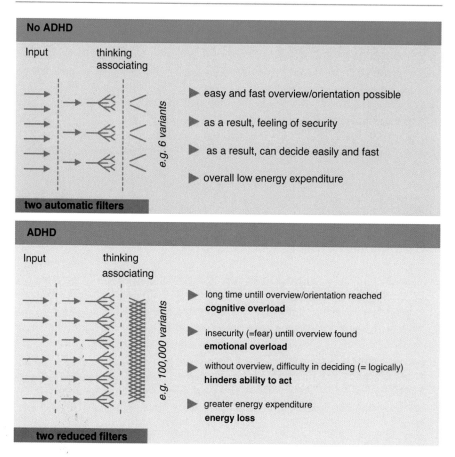

No ADHD

Input   thinking
         associating

e.g. 6 variants

▶ easy and fast overview/orientation possible

▶ as a result, feeling of security

▶ as a result, can decide easily and fast

▶ overall low energy expenditure

two automatic filters

ADHD

Input   thinking
         associating

e.g. 100,000 variants

▶ long time untill overview/orientation reached
  cognitive overload

▶ insecurity (=fear) untill overview found
  emotional overload

▶ without overview, difficulty in deciding (= logically)
  hinders ability to act

▶ greater energy expenditure
  energy loss

two reduced filters

Fig. 3.2 Filter and/or weighting model: the non-ADHD condition offers many advantages in everyday life/with the ADHD condition, much more information needs to be processed

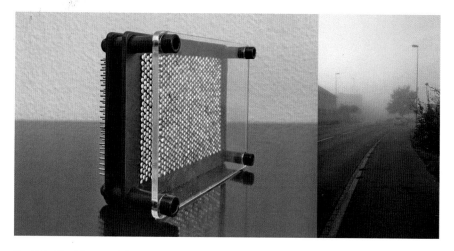

Fig. 3.3 Significance of the quantity of unweighted information: it is hard to differentiate because it is quasi at the same level ("like fog") → offers hardly any orientation

everyday life. This means that in unusual situations, fewer associations are available and new solution approaches are found only after a delay. This tends to be an obstacle to development and progress.

Conversely, ADHDers have an unchecked level of thinking, in comparison to non-ADHDers of the same intelligence. In everyday life, this can sometimes have confusing consequences, in line with "it's not that ADHDers think too little—they just think too widely". The overview of the unfiltered flood of data is easily lost, particularly the "perceived" overview. This isn't very practical for everyday tasks.

However, one veritable bonus does result from the minimal pre-filtering. It results in a larger breadth of association (Ryffel-Rawak 2017), more creative-innovative thinking and a greater willingness to follow new solution paths (Fig. 3.4).

Important: Although there is more information to process with ADHD, and it therefore takes longer in the default state until the ADHDer gets an overview or finds orientation, this does not at all mean that ADHDers are always slower. ADHDers are faster than comparable non-ADHDers under the following two conditions:

- In areas in which ADHDers have been working for a long time with interest, they are usually faster in recognising new circumstances and in finding a suitably adapted way to deal with them than comparable non-ADHDers. Imagine a taxi driver who has been working in the same city for 20 years and therefore is able to react particularly quickly and "intuitively" to different road conditions—it's the same thing.
- In an area in which an ADHDer has developed specific coping mechanisms, ADHDers can differentiate the important from the unimportant extremely quickly with the help of their well-trained coping mechanisms.

Encore
It's important to stress here: having possible difficulties with ADHD does not mean that "an ADHDer cannot do this" per se and permanently.

This is a phrase that one hears often, even among medical specialists. It's always important to take a look and see if a difficulty is actually caused by a lack of understanding of how you function, a lack of useful coping mechanisms or misunderstandings. Then you can adjust and learn to deal with the difficulty in another way. The boundaries are often not as narrow as you may think.

During this book, I will often refer to the basic form of the filter model. It is a concept which is easy to understand and offers fast initial usable insights, both into your own ADHD, if you have the condition, or observations into the behaviour of ADHDers. The more you can apply it in everyday life, the more benefit you will gain for living with ADHD. It's possible to understand most ADHD phenomena with it and gives you the opportunity to find constructive way of coping.

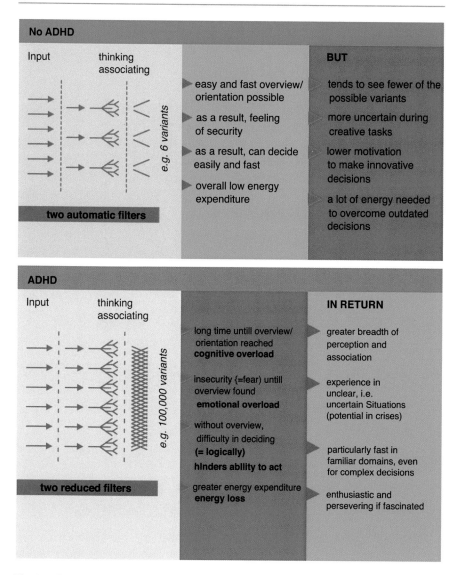

Fig. 3.4 Expanded filter model: the non-ADHD condition also has disadvantages; in return, the ADHD has advantages

3.2 Functions: Controlling and Dosing—The Control Model

The so-called executive functions (e.g. areas of concentration, perception, impulse control and organisational functions) are present in ADHD completely normally.

Contrary to the definition "attention deficit and hyperactivity disorder", there is *no* deficit in the *ability* to pay attention!

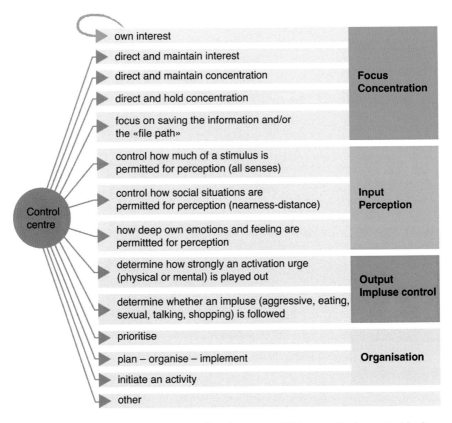

Fig. 3.5 Control model ADHD: executive functions are available normally, but control is situationally reduced (control centre less active); if the ADHDer is interested in a topic, the function is activated automatically

But the control centre that controls and doses these executive functions is less active (Barkley 1997; Brown 2005).

This can result in distractibility, concentration difficulties, perception disorders, hypersensitivity, hyperactivity, being scatter-brained, impulsiveness and organisational difficulties (Fig. 3.5).

In the following subchapters, you can find a description of what reduced control means for these functions individually, and what this reduced control can look like in everyday life.

3.2.1   Reduced Control in the Area of Focussing Functions: Concentration

3.2.1.1 Concentration and Distraction

If the control of the "concentration" function is less active, the logical consequence is rapid distraction. Everything which seems to be more interesting in that moment then captures the attention (Krause and Krause 2005). I would like to stress once again: ADHD is not a deficit in the ability to pay attention. It's just that the activation of the functions, which certainly are available, are linked to special prerequisites.

3.2.1.2 Hyperfocus: Positive and Negative is Possible
Particularly important:

- Similarly to the way that water flows down from a mountain, if there is only minimal control activity, the focus will shift by itself to the most interesting route.

   Although this is a disadvantage for less interesting work requiring continual concentration, it can be an advantage under certain circumstances. The concentration of an ADHDer is reliably focussed if they are directly currently interested in something, and **positive hyperfocus** is created (Hallowell and Ratey 1998). If this interest exists, ADHDers can concentrate better and for longer than non-ADHDers. This can represent one of the significant advantages of ADHD (see also Sects. 5.4 and 5.2.6).
- Reverse side of the coin: unfortunately the focus also shifts slightly wherever a stimulus disturbs, leading to **negative hyperfocus** (radical-negative situation and self-evaluation, correspondingly more extreme emotional and impulsive reactions, either defensively and/or self-accusatory-depressively). This is what causes a large proportion of suffering in ADHD (Figs. 3.6 and 3.7).

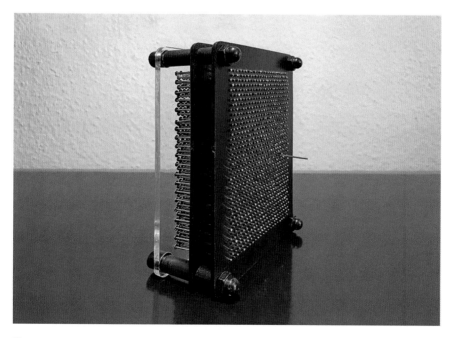

Fig. 3.6 Positive and negative hyperfocus: in the case of prominent, strong stimulus: own direct interest (fascination) → activation of concentration → positive hyperfocus; individual negative stimulus → activation of concentration → negative hyperfocus

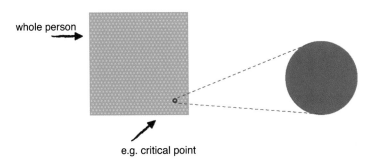

whole person

e.g. critical point

Objective reality
the entire value of the individual person is
contrasted with the small critical point

Subjective perception in negative hyperfocus
- I exist purely from this error
- and/or other people only see me in this way
- and/or other people are exclusively negative

Fig. 3.7 Negative hyperfocus (negative tunnel vision): perception is constricted (poss. totally) →
own value no longer perceived, therefore does not form a relativising counterbalance anymore

3.2.1.3 Negative Hyperfocus (Tunnel Vision): Quantitative

The negative hyperfocus (tunnel vision) described here leads above all to a *quantitative* intensification. Everything is enlarged, just like under a microscope. To put it in an extreme way (Fig. 3.7):

Situation	A mildly irritating remark is perceived as an absolutely unacceptable attack.
Emotional reaction	In an alleged unacceptable attack, the emotional reaction is not mild irritation but correspondingly intense anger.
Impulse to act	The resulting impulse to act therefore is not limited to a self-assured demarcation of boundaries, as would be appropriate as a reaction to a mildly irritating comment and mild annoyance. Instead it develops into an uncontrolled "seismic" counterattack and consequently into further, mutual escalation.

Through the hyperfocus, vision is indeed limited to the topic that provoked it in terms of content. But within this content, the thoughts and associations affected continue completely unchecked—and even uncontrolled.

This kind of negative tunnel vision is common. It is disastrous. So, it's even more important to learn how to deal with it. I will discuss this in more detail in Chap. 6.

3.2.1.4 Negative Hyperfocus (Tunnel Vision): Qualitative

In this form of hyperfocus, the meaning of the overall situation changes owing to the fact that the ADHDer's overview of the "big picture" is restricted. The content of the situation is fundamentally distorted and it appears to be a completely different situation.

Logically, the situation is evaluated according to the distorted perception; the emotional reaction and the action stimuli triggered both reflect the distortion. The

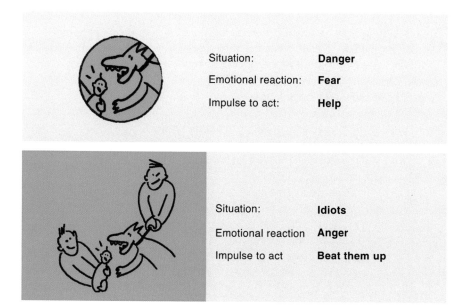

Fig. 3.8 Qualitative negative hyperfocus: when seeing things through tunnel vision (only part of the entire picture) distorts the meaning of the situation, the type of reaction also changes

entire substance regarding the quality of the overall situation is affected and not only the intensity of the perception and reaction.

In Fig. 3.8, in the tunnel vision view, there appears to be a situation in which a baby is about to be bitten in the head by a huge dog. This picture triggers a completely different reaction when compared to the entire picture. Here you see two guys grinning in a stupid way. One is holding the baby near the dog; the other is controlling the dog. There is no acute danger for the baby, but we cannot avoid thinking that the two guys are complete idiots.

I invented this crude example to demonstrate the principle of qualitative hyperfocus. So, I have included a case study (below) which shows how qualitative hyperfocus can occur in everyday life.

Case Study 2
The Doctor Who Was Almost Blind
A few years ago, I submitted a paper which was very important to me to a very renowned specialist journal. A week later I received the notice of receipt and that my essay had made it to the peer review process. In this process, renowned specialists write an appraisal of the article to decide whether it would be published or rejected.

After months of waiting, I received an email from the publisher which contained the phrase "MAJOR CHANGES HAVE TO BE MADE".

I was devasted—and really angry at the same time. I was on the point of ringing up the editorial office of the publisher to ask which idiots had been given my paper to review. But then I thought better of it. I remembered all the things I had already written about negative hyperfocus, including in the very article I had submitted to the journal.

So, I tried to calm down and take a closer look at the email. And those words did actually appear, but I had misread the context.

The email actually said, "We are happy to inform you that your paper is accepted for publication and that no major changes have to be made."

My tunnel vision had blanked out the decisive "no" and that changed the meaning of the message to the opposite of what was actually written.

3.2.1.5 Alleged Compulsion Problem

Setting the function "focus on saving a piece of information" is a considerable task in itself. This means that in ADHDers, the save function is not automatically activated when they listen attentively. Or—and this is significant—when they attentively perform a task.

This is particularly noticeable in routine actions. They *can* be performed attentively. But if the save function is not activated at the same time, you will not know afterwards what you have done and whether you actually did it.

An everyday phenomenon which is extremely common in ADHD is the following scenario: After breakfast, you switch off the coffee machine, turn off the lights and close the apartment door behind you. After a few steps, you ask yourself if you have done these things and check again. Several times. You find it embarrassing that you need to check this and become increasingly secretive about it because you are worried about being labelled an obsessive neurotic.

To make one thing absolutely clear: this has nothing to do with an obsessive-compulsive disorder (OCD). Even though the symptom appears to be similar. This is simply because in ADHDers, the function "save" is activated less automatically when carrying out routine actions. This ADHD-caused seemingly compulsive symptom is comparatively easy to overcome by training conscious ("manual") saving. This is totally in contrast to real obsessive-compulsive disorders which usually need intensive therapy.

Encore

By the way: the phenomenon of routine actions being saved less automatically plays a role in drug treatment for ADHDers, whether they are for ADHD or other conditions. If taking your medication becomes established, i.e. a routine action, it can happen that directly after taking it, you are not sure whether you have actually taken it. So, you take it again by mistake.

This can lead to an accidental overdose. In this case, it's easy to avoid overdosing by mistake. Either use a medicine dispenser or take the medication with the help of a mobile phone alarm.

3.2.2 Reduced Regulation in the Area of Input Functions: Perception

Input functions have to do with the information we take in or absorb. They regulate which stimuli from all our sensory functions are allowed to be perceived by us, and how much.

This is normally regulated according to the situation. For example, you might not notice much the pain of a powerful shove while intensively playing in a football match, but the same amount of pain after a relaxing sunbathing session even more.

In ADHD, this situational regulation can be slower, either in an upwards or a downwards direction, or even blocked. This means that ADHDers may be more sensitive in their reactions to sensory stimuli such as odours, light or noise—or, conversely, be almost completely impervious to them.

This alone can lead to difficulties at work, for example. If ADHDers react more strongly to odours such as stale sweat or perfume, they may be unjustly accused of reacting like the princess in Hans Christian Andersen's fairy-tale The Princess and the Pea. The same also applies to intense itching due to the label in your shirt. Or by contrast, it can lead to an ADHDer being suspected of having a hearing problem if acoustic stimuli are registered but perceived to a lesser extent.

In these situations, conflicts can quickly develop. It isn't necessarily the heightened or reduced perception that is the real problem but is much more likely to be the misunderstandings that result from them.

Case Study 3
The Postal Delivery Woman with the Bruises
Emma was about 50 years old. The misunderstandings that resulted from a reduced level of perception almost ruined her marriage. She had a reduced sensitivity to the pain of injuries or bumps. For many years, she had worked for the post office 1 day a week. Always doing the same job.

One evening, Emma's husband noticed bruises on the sides of both of her upper arms. He was concerned and asked her what happened. She had no idea, was ashamed and reacted a little flippantly. The same symptoms kept on reoccurring for several weeks, always after her day at work.

Emma increasingly resented her husband's questioning. He became mistrustful and began to suspect that she had a lover at work who was physically rough with her.

Understandably, Emma became even more angry and her husband became even more mistrustful.

Exactly at this point during her treatment, we spoke about the possible irregularities of perception with ADHD. Knowing about this helped Emma to see the situation less defensively: she was embarrassed that she didn't know what caused the bruises, which is why she had reacted indignantly.

With this special knowledge about the regulation of the perception sensory stimuli, Emma was able to have a certain amount of understanding for the suspicions of her husband—although he had also reacted not very smartly to the situation.

Now that she had acknowledged the issue, Emma was able to pay attention to how the bruises came to be on her arm.

The rest of the story is easily explained. It appeared that a new shelf had been put up in the post office behind a door that she always had to pass through during her day at work. In ADHD-style, Emma would hurry around this curve. In ADHD-style, her room orientation, which had become firmly established over the years, stayed the same.

The shelf was not calculated into this orientation. She therefore bumped into the shelf with her right arm in one direction, and with her left arm in the other direction—but didn't notice the pain. As she only worked once a week, the bruises could heal before the next bump. The pain wasn't particularly great, otherwise she would have noticed it and been able to adjust to the different room dimensions.

Ultimately, the problem wasn't the ADHD and the reduced level of perception, but the misunderstanding that arose from it.

It was good that Emma and also her husband were then able to laugh about the incident.

The input functions also include, in a wider sense, perception of one's own feelings and the understanding of social situations. Both play a large part in ADHD. I reflect on these functions in all chapters of this book.

3.2.3   Reduced Regulation in the Area of Output Functions: Impulse Control

Reduced impulse control, in association with physical hyperactivity, is one of the most well-known possible symptoms of ADHD (Bari and Robbins 2013). Or put another way: a stronger level of impulsiveness.

Here I would expressly like to point out that impulsiveness does not simply refer to aggressive impulses, as many people believe. This can happen, of course. But ADHDers tend to be rather peace-loving types. Even though many of them exhibited explosive temperaments in childhood, a substantial number of them learned to control this in time.

In the world of work, impulsiveness plays a role particularly in the impulse to speak. The regulation can take place either upwards or downwards.

Blocked impulse control when talking can lead to mental blocks and being impatient with the person you are talking to.

Giving in to the impulse in an uncontrolled way leads to a disruptive flood of speech, which gives little space to other people. This often leads to ADHDers impatiently interrupting their conversational partner. Impulsive reasoning, during which confidential information leaks out, can easily disrupt negotiation tactics during a business meeting. Many types of tension and misunderstandings can be caused in this way.

On the other hand, a reduced level of impulse control when speaking can also be the key to success. This is particularly the case in combination with a good level of intelligence and a wide association level. An above-average number of cabaret artists, journalists and television presenters are ADHDers.

It's also interesting to note that examinations have shown that in certain circumstances, impulsiveness can be an important factor in enabling entrepreneurs with ADHD to have commercial success (Wiklund et al. 2016).

What's more, reduced impulse regulation can also affect all other areas of life in which impulses play a role. This includes eating, in terms of both an increased and a reduced impulse to eat. Various eating disorders are more common with ADHD. Sexual impulses can also be affected. Impulsive buying behaviour can occur, as can obsessive gaming or addictive drug-taking. From a purely statistical perspective, ADHDers have a higher than average likelihood of developing an addiction. But we need to be careful here: a statistic is a statement about a collective group of people and says nothing at all about each individual in this collective. We know that addiction development is likely above all in those ADHDers who also have a social behaviour disorder (Modestin et al. 2001).

3.2.4 Reduced Control in the Area of Organisational Functions

Organisational matters play a large role in every kind of job. If it's possible for organisational functions such as prioritising, planning and implementation to be affected in ADHD, then this can have a major effect on an ADHDer's working life (Solden 1995).

Here the important word is "can"—not "must".

As I emphasised earlier, not every ADHDer is necessarily affected by all phenomena. Sometimes it's the case that ADHDers find the organisational tasks of their job easy—or even enjoyable! At the same time, the same people find it almost impossible to organise their private lives, neglect to plan their holidays, miss films that they would like to see or even forget the birthday of their spouses.

As an extreme example, I know a top female manager with ADHD who is perfectly organised in her job which includes coordinating meetings with decision-makers throughout the entire world, is always up-to-speed with her written reports, keeps her work desk tidy—and on the other hand, does not have her private affairs such as tax records, correspondence with authorities, organisation of insurances under control, nor can she keep on top of personal issues such as tidiness in her apartment or staying in touch with friends. This pattern is fairly common and means a lot of hidden misery to cope with.

In later chapters I will explore organisational issues connected with the world of work in more detail.

3.3   Coping: Profit, Side Effects and Misunderstandings

Overcoming or dealing with ADHD is described using the terms "coping" and "coping mechanisms". All ADHDers develop more or less useful strategies with which they can find their way in a world primarily made up of non-ADHDers:

- The attempt to find one's bearings in the flood of information and thoughts.
- The attempt to cope with the fact that the executive functions (concentration, perception, impulse control, organisation) are difficult to activate without certain prerequisites.

Please note: the development of these coping mechanisms begins very early in life. Young ADHD children do not know that in certain areas they function in a different way to the average child. Even if an ADHD diagnosis is made during the child's school years, an in-depth exploration of how ADHD works and what that means in everyday life only takes place in a very limited number of cases. The image is usually a distorted one and it is usually only the negative aspects that are perceived. This applies to the person affected and the people around them.

Under these prerequisites, the development of coping mechanisms requires a degree of effort that should not be underestimated.

Naturally, there are coping mechanisms that are constructive and effective, as well as those that tend to have an adverse effect. Constructive coping mechanisms can have side effects and lead to misunderstandings and difficulties too, both among family/friends/colleagues and the individual person concerned.

As in the illustration: some ADHDers find it difficult to select from a menu list in a restaurant. "Oh, there are so many possibilities! Is the fish here especially good or bad? What are the colleagues talking about? And those on the next table? Who's just walked in? Why is the music so loud?" Total confusion. For these everyday situations, there are numerous coping possibilities:

- I look at the menu beforehand on the internet and choose calmly at home
- I make a note of three dishes that I like and of which I can expect that at least one of them will be on the menu in every restaurant; then I choose that one
- I always choose the same as the other person
- etc.

Each of these coping strategies works to some extent.
Each has its own side effects.
If I always order the same as the other person, I will probably not be eating what I really like for a lot of the time. A small price to pay to avoid the agony of choice. It will be worse if the other person gets the impression that I don't have my own opinion. Both on a date or during a business lunch with the boss, the chances of a

promotion will sink. But the worst thing is if you're not sure why you have problems choosing from the menu. Then you begin to doubt yourself and regard yourself as a slowcoach. You become insecure and defensive.

Side effects and misunderstandings like these cause a large proportion of the suffering in ADHD. They are an unnecessary kind of collateral damage. A collateral damage that can often be easily prevented.

If the ADHDer in the above example is clear about why he has problems with choosing from the menu, then he doesn't doubt his self-worth. He recognises it as being a relatively unimportant consequence of his way of functioning which is beneficial to him in more important areas of his life (e.g. imaginative working).

With this new feeling of self-assurance, achieved through knowledge of his ADHD, he can use the same coping mechanism, but proactively, thereby avoiding numerous side effects. So now he says to his boss, "I want to be able to concentrate fully on our discussion, and not be preoccupied with the menu, so I'll have the same as you." In this way he positions himself as someone who definitely makes his own decisions. And who knows what is important to him: here, the discussion with his boss.

Encore

It's well worth trying to work out how to classify your own personal ADHD-related difficulties as much as possible.

- Which difficulties are primary ADHD phenomena, i.e. they have a direct neurobiological cause.
- Which are secondary phenomena, i.e. unhelpful coping mechanisms, side effects of helpful coping mechanisms and misunderstandings.
- Which are long-term developments, long-term consequences.

This differentiation is decisive in weighting the phenomenon according to the individual situation, and in putting together the therapeutic treatment. In which situations does medication help? And for which situation or when could medication be counterproductive? In which context is it particularly important to communicate information about ADHD? Under what prerequisites would cognitive, systemic or psychodynamic psychotherapy approaches be promising—or a hindrance? in which areas can structures and technical aids be helpful?

When I write about the choosing therapeutic treatment here, then I am referring not just to the physicians and psychotherapists, but also to ADHDers themselves. On the one hand, as an encouragement to get involved in managing their own treatment, and on the other, in their own everyday reflections on how they handle their ADHD in that moment.

References

Armstrong CL, Hayes KM, Martin R. Neurocognitive problems in attention deficit disorder. Alternative concepts and evidence for impairment in inhibition of selective attention. Ann NY Acad Sci. 2001;931:196–215.

Bari A, Robbins TW. Inhibition and impulsivity: behavioral and neural basis of response control. Prog Neurobiol. 2013;108:44–79.

Barkley RA. Behavioral inhibition, sustained attention, and executive functions: constructing a unifying theory of ADHD. Psychol Bull. 1997;121:65–94.

Brown TE. Attention-deficit disorder: the unfocused mind in children and adults. New Haven, CT: Yale University Press; 2005.

Faraone S. A family genetic perspective. New York: APA; 2004.

Hallowell EM, Ratey JJ. Zwanghaft zerstreut. Reinbeck: Rowohlt; 1998.

Krause J, Krause KH. ADHS im Erwachsenenalter. Stuttgart, New York: Schattauer; 2005.

Modestin J, Matutat B, Würmle O. Antecedents of opioid dependence and personality disorder: attention-deficit/hyperactivity disorder and conduct disorder. Eur Arch Psychiatry Clin Neurosci. 2001;251:42–7.

Ryffel-Rawak D. Unser facettenreiches Leben. Hamburg: Verlag tredition; 2017.

Solden S. Women with attention-deficit disorder. Embracing disorganization at home and in the workplace. Grass Valley: Underwood Books; 1995.

Stieglitz RD, Hofecker-Fallahpour M. Workshop "ADHS bei Erwachsenen". Winterthur; 2007.

Trott GE. Das hyperkinetische Syndrom und seine medikamentöse Behandlung. Leipzig: Johann Ambrosius Barth; 1993.

Wiklund J, Patzelt H, Dimov D. Entrepreneurship and psychological disorder: how ADHD can be productively harnessed. J Bus Ventur Insights. 2016;6:14–20.

Fundamentals of ADHD in the World of Work

4

4.1 To Come Out or Not?

The question often arises as to whether an ADHDer should "come out" about the condition at work. There is no generally valid answer here because it depends very much on the individual circumstances. Nevertheless, I would like to present a few aspects which may help you to make the decision:

4.1.1 Don't Be Over Hasty: Beware of Prejudices

Once you've published the information, you can't ever take it back. If you tell people too soon about your diagnosis, you risk being pigeonholed as a troublemaker. Don't forget that ADHD can also be seen as a "completely natural 'wiring' of the brain" (quote from Weiss 1996).

As a general rule, the label ADHD shouldn't be the first priority during a job interview. You are likely to come across too many prejudices and too little knowledge of the facts. The idea of a job application is to make the initial contact, create the initial basis for a professional relationship, present your own qualities and get further information about the job and the company. It is usually not appropriate to give out sensitive information.

However, it is sensible to give out the information at an early stage if you will be relying on the employer making substantial allowances in the working conditions, owing to your ADHD-related idiosyncrasies (see Sect. 9.2.5).

The same usually applies for the initial period of working in a new job.

© The Author(s), under exclusive license to Springer Nature Switzerland AG 2023
H. Lachenmeier, *ADHD and Success at Work*,
https://doi.org/10.1007/978-3-031-13437-1_4

4.1.2   Functional Pattern: Problem-Free Coming Out—Initially Without "ADHD" Label

There's plenty you can say about ADHD as a functional pattern—in other words, how you tick, *without* mentioning the diagnosis by name. It includes talking about possible difficulties, but also the advantages. Later, when some common ground has been established, you always have the option of using the diagnosis term—the label ADHD.

4.1.3   Honesty Is Not the Same as Oversharing

It's important not to confuse being honest with "oversharing" or a kind of non-stop verbal "incontinence". In the same way, openness/transparency shouldn't be confused with exhibitionism.

Honesty means neither lying nor deceiving but, at the same time, keeping the decision about what personal information you divulge to others, under your own control. In the same way, transparency does not mean that others have an entitlement to your private life. The terms transparency and openness should also not be misused to justify always putting yourself and your ego in the limelight.

> **Encore**
> Many ADHDers are excessively open and honest in a way which is actually self-sabotaging. Here I am not suggesting that this is an unconscious "wanted" urge to self-sabotage (as is the case in so-called neurotic superego pathologies). In ADHD, it's much more a case of an accidental exaggerated honesty/openness, whether it is through a reduced impulse control or a coping mechanism when a fog of information and thought leads to the ADHDer losing sight of the big picture.
>
> Don't forget: the desire for a private sphere is absolutely normal, healthy and appropriate—it has absolutely nothing to do with a lack of transparency.
> (see also Sect. 4.2.4).

In a job application, the only important thing is that I improve my chances of being offered the position I desire, and that I check my suitability for the company (and vice-versa). It's not the time to explain to the public about ADHD or start a de-stigmatisation campaign.

> **Encore**
> Outings of an ADHD diagnosis in the context of public information and de-stigmatisation campaigns should be carried out by people who would not suffer any disadvantage from coming out, e.g. young celebrities from the worlds of business, sport and culture. Or also older professionals who have established themselves in ordinary professions and whom "no one can touch any more" such as a psychiatrist who has his own practice.

Whether and when you now come out, or not, it's worthwhile keeping the following orientation point ("fixed star") in mind:

I'm not perfect—but all the others are not perfect either.

4.2   ADHD: Who Am I at Work?

4.2.1   Be Careful with One-Sided Generalisations About ADHD

There isn't a clearly defined "model" of the working person with ADHD. It's important to beware of generalisations such as "ADHDers can't work in open-plan offices because they are too easily distracted". Sweeping absolutisms like this can unnecessarily narrow your room for manoeuvre.

4.2.1.1 Distracted by External Stimuli
For example, the limitation regarding open-plan offices only applies for those ADHDers in which the sensory overload is primarily triggered by the unfiltered assimilating of external stimuli.

4.2.1.2 Distracted by Internal Stimuli
For those ADHDers in which the sensory overload primarily occurs through their own flood of thoughts, an open-plan office or the background noise in a busy restaurant can even help to put the brakes on the side branches of the too widely associating thinking to such an extent that the distractibility is reduced. This means that the ADHDer is better able to concentrate on the task to be carried out. Some top journalists with ADHD only function in this way (Fig. 4.1).

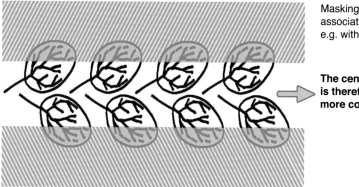

Masking the too widely associating thinking, e.g. with noise

The centre is therefore more concentrated

Fig. 4.1 Background noises can sometimes even help you to concentrate

4.2.2 How Does My ADHD Function and How Do *I Myself* Handle It

As you follow your professional path with ADHD, it's not only important to consider your interests and talents—and thereby the fact that you have ADHD. The main issue is how you handle your ADHD: constructively or with behavioural patterns that are less useful?

Therefore, a central issue is: how can I learn to handle my ADHD constructively, when I understand how it functions?

> **Encore**
> Ways of coping with ADHD can differ greatly. The effects can be correspondingly different—and even contradictory. Mostly these coping mechanisms are not conscious, because you have developed them early in your life.

Here is a small selection of negative examples which can create different life paths in comparably talented ADHDers. This depends on individual coping methods, different ways of handling too much information and thoughts, an inability to "see the big picture" and difficulties in making decisions.

- In order not to have to make a decision, I simply take on all tasks, help my colleagues, do overtime, learn an enormous amount doing it, hope that it's enough, but nevertheless am regarded as being inefficient because I neglect my own core tasks and ultimately become exhausted.
- I have many ideas but am doubtful whether they are well thought through and/or whether I have understood the issue in the first place, which was possibly meant in a different way to the way I thought. I always hold back, owing to my uncertainty, express my ideas during the coffee break; these are then implemented by others leading to me feeling exploited, not appreciated enough and I become resentful.
- So as not to get lost in all the data, thoughts and decisions, I choose a job which is easy and monotonous, offering me limited room to manoeuvre; where I can do my job according to the rules (without needing to think). This means that I am never under pressure, feel safe, do not develop my potential any further, but initially feel very content. But it's quite common that sooner or later, the feeling of having missed out on something emerges.
- I lose myself in inner worlds, drift off into daydreams and therefore do not feel any stress...for the moment. This can be a constructive way of coping, if I only use it for a short time, a momentary stabilisation. But it can also lead to me feeling that I'm inefficient, even for simple jobs and that I have got bogged down in terms of my career.
- To get an overall view of everything, I go in search of the adrenalin kick that enables me to focus and organise all the data, and under which I can display my

best abilities. This means that I am continually in a hurry, always looking for something new, restless, shift between top fit and collapsed with exhaustion, between being overconfident and insecure. In the best-case scenario, I thereby have an exciting life; in the worst case, early total burnout.

Some of these examples reveal a readiness to show modesty and self-sacrifice, or a willing dedication to others. In all of them, it's possible to recognise an honest attempt to somehow live up to the demands of life. Nevertheless, the examples selected show the typical strained ADHD life paths. A decisive number of these strains result from coping with ADHD. This coping mechanism was shaped by the persons affected, owing to lack of knowledge about ADHD, in a way that has led to negative consequences, despite all efforts to the contrary.

This can largely be prevented, if the right knowledge is there.

4.2.3   Hierarchy, Office Politics and Apparent Naivety

ADHDers—particularly the intelligent ones—often seem to be strangely naive. Spirited, worldly, confident—and like an innocent country bumpkin at the same time. This can have a devastating impact when dealing with hierarchies and office politics.

Although this seems to be contradictory, there is a certain logic behind it:

- Let's keep the basic configuration of ADHD in mind, with too much unfiltered information from outside and too many unchecked own thoughts as well. If we want to make sense of this flood of data, then it's a good idea not to complicate things unnecessarily. In other words: it is completely understandable that one eagerly assumes that everything in this world is straightforward. As straightforward as it is for small children (which is the age at which many of the ADHD coping mechanisms are developed). This means that one simply holds onto the "straightforwardness" as a form of coping, because double or multiple meaning would allow the combination of possibilities to grow exponentially, whereby even the most capable brain would be quickly overloaded in terms of quantity.
- Strictly speaking, it's not really about naivety in the narrow sense, but about a coping mechanism with the aim of keeping the amount of processing that the brain needs to do to a more or less manageable quantity.

Encore
Every normal intelligent ADHDer has experienced thousands of times the fact that this kind of coping—assuming the world is straightforward—doesn't work very well. However, we often don't consider personal coping mechanisms as being problematic. Mostly we don't even recognise them. It's much more likely that we will complain about the dishonesty of the world. It's true that there is a lot of malicious dishonesty, but there's also a kind of natural ambiguity which no-one is to blame for and even has its roots in the core of human life. Just think of flirting, for instance.

After finishing an apprenticeship, for example: you start a new job, want to prove yourself and do your very best. After a while, you become skilled and well versed in your tasks, are pleased with yourself and hope that your superiors will reward your good performance appropriately. You are particularly hopeful of getting the relevant encouragement from your direct superior, who sometimes appears to be out of his depth and whom you have "bailed out" several times. So why does he send your obviously less competent office partner to the exciting advanced-training seminar while fobbing you off with the boring unskilled jobs?

This is clearly unfair. And how can one possibly understand it? The boss should leave!—only, in the end, it is you yourself that end up leaving.

The sequence of events described here happens all the time. Even to non-ADHDers. And even some of these don't understand why. It's just that non-ADHDers usually recognise it in early adulthood as a reality that is ambiguous, peculiar and unfair, but that one simply has to come to terms with.

By contrast, ADHDers are in danger of either pursuing fruitless head-on confrontations or sinking into a mood of resignation and depression at an early stage.

It therefore logically follows that if you have ADHD, it's even more important to learn how hierarchies and office politics work. It's not necessary to find these rules great (because they're not, anyway), but you need to be aware of them, because otherwise you'll be lost. In the same way: if you go on a ski tour without an awareness of avalanches, you'll soon be buried under the snow. Avalanches are definitely not great; but ski tours are great, as long as you are *not* buried under an avalanche.

Encore

Here are a few details about the example quoted above of an employee who was overlooked and ultimately dismissed. Insights from the classic book "The Peter Principle" (Peter and Hull 1969), which describes how hierarchies function in the world of work are useful in explaining this case. I recommend this slim and extremely entertaining little book for every ADHDer.

The most well-known conclusion is that everyone is promoted until they reach a point at which they are no longer competent. It's important to note that the law of the Peter Principle only applies in complex hierarchies with several hierarchy levels. But here it proves to be reliable, whether it is a philanthropic organisation or a multinational arms-smuggling syndicate.

On this basis, it's clear that a superior who has already reached this end point, is usually not very pleased about having a capable and enthusiastic subordinate, because this triggers his fear of competition. Consequently, he suppresses the capable employee but not the incapable one, who doesn't represent a threat to him.

Those who are not so interested in reading non-fiction books can read about the laws of hierarchies and office politics in the novel "Something Happened" (Heller 1974). It's also a brilliant book, but longer and also cynical in parts.

With the Peter Principle too, it's important to beware of generalisations in absolute terms: not every superior who doesn't like you has necessarily already reached the "point of his own incompetence" (see "The Peter Principle"). There are thousands of factors on both sides, which can cause rejection.

4.2.4 Are There Questions to Be Answered Here?

Worth mentioning as a variant for the apparent naivety mentioned in Sect. 4.2.3 is the issue of how ADHDers deal with questions that they are asked. In order to reduce the excess of discernible possibilities when asked a question, ADHDers tend often—for the sake of simplicity—simply not to scrutinise the questions.

This even occurs—sometimes more than ever—with ADHDers who otherwise tend to question everything and everyone, and who cannot allow any statement to go unchallenged. But the aforementioned simplification appears here in a covert way.

Namely:

If these ADHDers are asked a question, then they automatically give an answer.

If I speak to these types of ADHDers about this, then they usually look at me in pure astonishment or even blankly.

Patient	"But of course I'm giving an answer. You asked a question!"
HL	"And when I ask what colour your underpants are?"
Patient	"Black, because you see..."
HL	"I didn't ask the question because I wanted to know the answer. But for another reason. Because let's be honest: it's none of my business what colour your underpants are."
Patient	"Oh, yes, that's true!"

A great deal of insight can be acquired as a result.

- Firstly about how to understand the coping mechanism of the automatic answer.
- Secondly about the banal things of human existence that can be of great significance in the world of work. Banal things that quite often even very intelligent ADHDers are completely unaware of.

 Such as the fact that questions can be asked not only to get a relevant answer, but for thousands of other reasons.

After their first amazement, they painfully remember many such situations in which they had to make embarrassing moves to explain themselves, allowed themselves to be forced onto a defensive footing, held seemingly responsible for the mistakes of others, were pressured into taking on additional tasks or simply put their foot in it in some way.

The realisation that this stems not from alleged stupidity but as the effect of an early developed, plausible coping mechanism with ADHD, is a great relief.

Above all because it shows that there is the possibility to change. Most intelligent ADHDers develop an almost Sherlock Holmes-like investigative delight in discovering how questions can be considered. In a certain sense, an additional dimension in understanding themselves *and* their surroundings emerges.

And naturally, it's also about acquiring ADHD-suitable means of orientation, both for the classification of questions as well as selecting one's own reaction.

Suggested Solutions to Dealing with Questions

4.2.4.1 As a Rough Guide
Is the question…

- … justified in terms of content
- … made with a constructive attitude
- … in an appropriate context
- … and asked by a qualified person?
- Or are there indications of a conscious or unconscious hidden agenda?

If the first four points can be answered with "yes" and the last with "no", then a direct content-related answer is usually a good idea.

4.2.4.2 About the Differentiated Assessment
Otherwise you will need to ask yourself a few questions to be able to make a precise assessment of the situation. For example:

- Do I even allow the other person to ask this question?
- In what form do the context and content of the question differ from one another (important information in passing; confidential chat in the canteen; private talk in an official meetings; etc.)?
- Does the other party want to put me under pressure?
- Is the purpose of the question to lead me "up the garden path"?
- Is the person asking the question feigning ignorance to sway me into security?
- Is the person asking the question feigning weakness and vulnerability, to mislead me into supporting him?
- And so on.

4.2.4.3 Choosing a Possible Reaction
There are also countless possible types of reaction available. For example:

- Simply ignore the question and skip it
- Answer with a counterquestion yourself
- An ironic, sarcastic or even cynical remark as a reaction
- Call into question whether the person has a right to ask this question
- Verbally attack the questioner
- Leave the person asking the question uncertain with statements that slightly avoid the question, are correct in terms of content but that say nothing

- Mislead the person asking the question with a tactical lie
- And so on

Keep the different variations in mind. It's worth practising them. First in your head only, and then in insignificant situations. Finally in a serious situation where it plays a role.

These tips should be sufficient here. I am sure that as soon as they recognise the basic principle, everyone will be able to apply it in given time. There is also plenty of literature out there on the topic of rhetoric, the art of debating and negotiation tactics. Observations made during media training seminars can also be very enlightening in this context.

The phenomenon of the over-adapted naive answer can naturally also be found—like many other phenomena described here—in non-ADHDers, although by no means as often. In these cases, the problem is often more complex and cannot be remedied by simple means.

4.2.5   Social Life and Small Talk at Work

Some ADHDers are charm personified. At a very early age, they have already absorbed all direct visible forms of social interaction in an unfiltered way. Moreover, they have grasped with which of these forms they can achieve favourable reactions. They manoeuvre themselves in everyday social interactions like a fish gliding through water.

We are envious of them because these abilities to charm are well-known to be extremely helpful in everyday working life.

> **Encore**
> To avoid misunderstandings, I would like to stress: be wary of equating these abilities in everyday social interaction with the ability to have problem-free relationships on all levels. ADHDers with a perfect charming, self-assured appearance can also be battling feelings of inner self-doubt or have difficulties with emotional closeness.

A very large number of ADHDers tend to have difficulties with everyday interactions, however.

It's true that non-ADHDers don't always find this easy too. Young people particularly often go through an absolutist-idealistic phase of total rejection of society's conventions during adolescence such as enquiring about health or small talk. Both are vilified as being phony and superficial: "*if someone, asked how they were doing, replied that they were doing badly, everyone would be embarrassed. Small talk is only for superficial people who have no depth, don't know what to say and who are self-sufficiently looking for mutual confirmation in their respective social class*".

Most non-ADHDers lose this attitude early during their adult lives. The societal function of small talk and similar customs is at the very least acknowledged.

ADHDer however often continue to hold the opinion that this convention is superficial, dishonest and should be rejected. To accept it would mean taking ambiguity into consideration, and thereby the thought trees would become even larger.

The rejection of such conventions is therefore a further variant by which the quantity of the thoughts to be processed is reduced by automatic simplification. In other words, to take things simply at face value, literally, for the sake of simplicity.

Encore

Taking conventions and statements at face value, i.e. literally, is a characteristic that is typical of people with a personality on the autism spectrum (Riedel 2013). It can often be observed in people with ADHD too. In recent years it has been recognised that, contrary to earlier beliefs, ADHD and high-functioning autism can indeed occur simultaneously and exhibit several overlaps. There are hints that they are both based on the same genes. Research will probably be able to clarify this in the not-too-distant future.

In any case, it's interesting to see that the "literal" aspect can be observed in ADHD in the context of coping with the overlarge dose of data, as an attempt to simplify the world. One could therefore formulate the hypothesis that high-functioning autism may be a special form of coping that exhibits an ADHD structure. If we consider further phenomena and the ways in which ADHD and autism function, then there is a vast and not very well-explored field of research that promises to be endlessly exciting and beneficial to discover.

Back to ADHD. Like all coping mechanisms, the taking-everything-literally trait can have side effects. In this case, there are substantial limitations in social situations that often occur, in both professional and private life.

The good thing, however, is that most ADHDers quickly understand these contexts if they are explained to them. The disadvantageous taking-everything-literally trait can then be abandoned.

Suggested Solutions If You Find Small Talk Troublesome

4.2.5.1 First Step: Emotional

As so often with ADHD however, it's not about understanding something intellectually but creating the emotional prerequisite for implementing what you have perceived.

It's important that the person affected really understands that their simplification mechanism of taking everything literally has nothing to do with being stupid or intellectually slow. It is much more an expression of the creativity with which they try to deal with the flood of data from an early age, under prerequisites of which they were unaware.

So, it's very much an achievement to be proud of.

It's only the combination of the understanding and the feeling of pride that releases the willingness to call into question the coping mechanism used up to now.

> **Encore**
> Nota bene: the perception of this justified pride, the emotional recognition of one's own value, is required here. This is because in ADHD, many of the secondary difficulties are related to the, partly hidden, doubt in one's own worth. Self-doubt that blocks the implementation of intellectual reasoning.
>
> And vice-versa: a feeling of justified pride which, only now, releases the readiness for intellectual understanding and the implementation of the reasoning.
>
> (see also Chap. 6).

4.2.5.2 Second Step: Cognitive

If the first step has succeeded, then the basis for the second step is emotionally created. The rest is easy, because cognitively there's nothing much to understand. In brief:

- Everyone feels uncertainty and fear in social contacts. Above all when you meet someone again after not seeing them for a long time, or even more so when meeting new people. This applies even more when it concerns a large group of people. It's inevitable that we feel uncertain about the situation, because we don't yet know anything about the others. In this situation, the greeting is the little sister of small talk.
- In these kinds of situations, pleasantries such as "how are you doing?" have the exclusive function of breaking the ice between two people. Nothing more. Pleasantries are therefore the first step along a path that afterwards is perhaps already over, or can lead up the highest mountains. To answer this clichéd question about your health with the pleasantry "good" does not mean that you are being superficial but that you are showing consideration in saving your conversation partner from an embarrassing situation. Similarly, to bypass a more in-depth answer to the question about your health does not necessarily mean a lack of interest, but signals a respect for the private sphere of the other.
- The same goes for extended small talk. Its *function* is to enable people to talk to each other despite feeling uncertain, to get closer minimally or also perhaps only to temporarily fill in time until a business meeting begins.

  The most important thing about small talk is that absolutely all topics which could have a further significance for any of those present are *initially* absolutely forbidden.

  It is therefore not the weakness of small talk, that it doesn't say anything, but it is its most important and most valuable characteristic. It prevents disagreements before minimal contact has even occurred.

It's simple to implement this cognitively: the weather, the season, current public holidays and catastrophes are innocuous and make classic conversation topics. Political, religious, familial and amorous topics are tabu.

Any ADHDer can implement this, because suddenly you're no longer faced with an actual unsolvable task such as how to begin a deep and earth-shattering discussion within seconds. You know that you have absolutely nothing to prove. The primary aim of small talk is to identify something absolutely harmless, that is—if possible—*not* original. Then you can concoct two or three standard remarks about it. One of these remarks will always fulfil this minimal function.

Encore
In the everyday worlds of business and politics, there is also a further form of small talk that serves other goals: intrigues and so-called hidden agendas. These follow similar intentions to those described in the section on office politics. The purpose is to lure the other person into a trap: to unsettle him before a negotiation round, to spread rumours, to present oneself as allegedly harmless in order to reduce his alertness for the following session, and much more.

Naturally you can also learn this if you have the motivation to do so. Independent of ADHD. From the ADHD side, it's first about acquiring a balance between:

1. Banal small talk, extremely easy to deal with.
   Enables you to have a degree of composure and thereby decisively expands your own room for manoeuvre. Fundamentally constructive.
2. Entire range of negotiating and political intrigues that also occur in small talk. Quasi, the Machiavellian specialist training in negotiation techniques. Can be useful but also destructive. Requires substantial effort to learn.
   It is not absolutely necessary to master these intrigues. For most working professionals, it is really sufficient if you are aware of them without needing to examine them in detail. This is enough to stop you falling into traps.

4.2.6 Sleepless "Offside" at Work

Humans need sleep. It's hard to get through the day without enough sleep. This always affects a person's work activities. Quality and productivity decrease. Overtiredness dampens your mood; your patience is reduced—something which is particularly tricky in ADHD with its reduced impulse control. Professional relationships can suffer. And ultimately, all this can have an effect on your career.

ADHDers who sleep well do exist. They can fall asleep anywhere, at any time. They are to be envied.

Nevertheless, many ADHDers struggle a lot with sleep. They have endless stories of misery. It's a problem which should be taken seriously, and it doesn't just affect ADHDers. These days, an independent specialist field of medicine explores the issue of sleep and sleep problems.

In this book I will discuss several ADHD-specific tips. If the situations described below apply to you, the effect of them can be impressive. In the event of sleep problems of a different kind, unfortunately not.

4.2.6.1 Exciting and/or Annoying Chains of Association When Falling Asleep

Many ADHDers report that when falling asleep, all kinds of thoughts go through their heads—they have difficulty "switching off" (Schlösser 2006): new ideas, to-do lists or thoughts about the experiences of the previous day. The flood of these thought associations always includes something that is either fascinating enough or annoying enough to prevent the person affected from falling asleep.

It's clear that this mechanism is a direct effect of unchecked, unfiltered thinking.

Encore

Be careful: this phenomenon that affects some people is spontaneously referred to as "revolving thoughts". It's only after precise questioning that the variety of different thoughts on different topics are discovered: both positive and negative, most of them are directly related to events of the past or the coming day, meaning that they demonstrate a substantial variation over time.

This is not the same as "thinking in circles" which occurs as a psychopathological symptom, e.g. a depression and can be described as the tortuous revolving of the same content again and again, night after night. It's important that anyone affected knows this, because unfortunately there are quite a few specialists who, when confronted with terms such as "thinking in circles" or "revolving thoughts" don't ask precisely what is meant and automatically/algorithmically classify the problem as depression.

It's therefore a good idea to avoid general psychological and psychiatric specialist terms when you are speaking to someone like me. Simply use everyday language to describe your situation. Describe! Please openly declare possible interpretations to be just that: an interpretation. Then the likelihood of misunderstandings is reduced and there will be no automatic adoption of interpretations.

Many of the difficulties in falling asleep in ADHD result from these wide, sometimes exciting and sometimes annoying chains of association. The following story illustrates the basic principle of how to deal with them:

Case Study 4

The Man Who Was Ashamed of Sleeping Well

Matthias was a married man in his mid-thirties who had recently been diagnosed with ADHD. Although he knew that he had ADHD, he didn't yet know anything about it apart from a long list of negative symptoms. He got in touch because he wanted to know more about ADHD. During our conversations I mentioned that not all ADHDers had problems in open-plan offices (cf. Sect. 4.2.1). Some were able to work there particularly well because the many noises occupied their brain, meaning that their thinking was not filled with too wide associations. They ended up by being less restless and stayed concentrated.

On hearing this Matthias sat bolt upright and said that suddenly something was rather clear to him.

He had always had difficulties in falling asleep, even as a young boy. But he always felt drowsy and fell easily asleep when his mother did the vacuum cleaning. With time, he used the opportunity to have a sleep every time his mother brought out the vacuum cleaner.

When he moved out of his parental home to do his apprenticeship, he had the idea of using a hair drier which produced a similar sound. He constructed a holder for the hair drier, switched it on "cold", connected it to the electricity supply via a timer switch and was able to fall asleep splendidly.

Until he got a girlfriend.

When she came to visit, he hid the gadget, filled with shame, under his bed. The relationship progressed and after a while the two of them wanted to get married. Matthias knew that he could not and did not want to forgo his hair drier sleep permanently. With a heavy heart he made his fiancé promise not to tell anyone, not even her best friend, anything about his falling asleep gadget. She loved him, respected his wish, promised not to say anything and kept her promise for many years. In their everyday routine, he would go to bed 10 min earlier than his wife and as soon as the hair drier switched off, his wife joined him.

Matthias now explained that he not only understood why the hair drier was so helpful when he was falling asleep. It also became clear to him that there was absolutely no reason for him to be ashamed of his falling asleep gadget. On the contrary, it was an inspired solution.

We talked about this realisation from all possible perspectives. It was definitely inspired that, without knowing the slightest about the background reasons, he was able to correctly categorise an observation as a small boy and ultimately invent an absolutely harmless method to treat his sleep disorder. This realisation, this sensing of his own value, was doubly important. For years, he had been ashamed of his falling asleep technique.

It didn't take 2 weeks until Matthias had told all his friends, relatives and acquaintances about his falling asleep gadget. But with a chest justifiably swollen with pride.

Suggested Solutions for ADHD Sleep

This case study illustrates the way in which these ADHD-induced difficulties in falling asleep can be approached. Naturally it doesn't always help. And hair drier noises don't help everyone fall asleep, in any case. It's also possible to be so annoyed by these noises, that you cannot fall asleep at all.

So, it's about finding something that occupies your own brain to the extent that you concentrate on it a little (not more!), and that it distracts you enough so that your associations do not get too wide and out of hand.

Rain sounds help one person, other falls asleep to psychedelic music whereas this would make a third sit bolt upright in bed. Audio books are a proven method, although the stories should be ones that you know already. Otherwise, you may be stay awake out of a fear of missing something. My oldest and best friend, an ADHDer of the restless type, was able to sleep really well for the first time when he was sent, in the 1980s, with a delegation from his bank to a meeting in Chicago. The permanent traffic noises spiced with the occasional revving of engines, the different sirens and other typical sounds of an American metropolis rocked him into a blissful sleep. Whereas his colleagues turned up to the meeting the next morning feeling exhausted, he was better rested than ever before.

4.2.6.2 Non-pharmaceutical Stimulation for Falling Asleep

Stimulating yourself in order to fall asleep sounds like a paradox at first. But we remember: with ADHD, the automatic pre-filter is less active, meaning that thoughts can fly unfiltered and unchecked in all directions. A factor which can lead to difficulties in falling asleep, as described above. Moderate stimulation that is sufficient to activate the filter a little but not strongly enough to case general stimulation can be helpful here.

If you rinse your feet and calves with cold water directly before going to bed, then you activate a neuronal system that—for a few minutes—has a similar kind of activating effect. The decisive factor is that you must lie down to sleep straight after the rinsing. It works for a few lucky people.

Encore

And vice versa, it's important to bear in mind that in the case of possible drug-stimulant treatment, the effect doesn't just subside when you go to bed.

At this time, the so-called rebound phenomenon (Carlson and Kelly 2003) can easily occur in which the ADHD symptomatic is increased for 20–30 min or longer in certain circumstances. This makes falling asleep even harder.

In these cases, it's important to make sure that there is sufficient time between the sinking of the effect and going to bed (1–2 h). Or as a second variation, that the effect first falls under the threshold level when you have fallen asleep. The latter should remain the exception, however.

4.2.6.3 ADHD-Independent Tips on Sleeping

Naturally the usual recommendations for good sleeping habits (known as "sleep hygiene") also apply with ADHD. No blue computer light before going to bed, no hectic sending of emails, surfing, gaming or similar; a ritualised procedure, to some extent, for going to bed; rather cool and fresh air in the bedroom.

And one thing in particular: NO problem or problem-solving discussions before going to sleep. These kinds of discussion *at this time of day* have two consequences which occur almost without exception.

- The problems become larger not smaller; a possible conflict then runs the high risk of escalating
- You certainly won't be able to sleep afterwards

Rejecting these kinds of discussion *at this time of day* has nothing to do with refusing to discuss things in general. It's much more a case of necessary protection from guaranteed escalation.

Of course, it's important to aim to achieve this protective agreement not first as midnight approaches but during some other quiet point during the day. Regard it as a general preventative approach for these kinds of situations—for all couples.

And of course, people are different. Sometimes the opposite of that which is recommended turns out to be effective for a particular individual. What counts is a person's reality, not the general rule.

4.2.7   A Top Career Is Not Compulsory

At this point, I would like to point out something which is self-evident but, as is often the case with things that are self-evident, is easy to forget.

This book is about being successful in your job with ADHD. Successful is often equated with winning a competition. Of course, the winner's position is a success position. But it is just one of several. And even a victory can be a failure, for example in the form of a Pyrrhic victory (although King Pyrrhus won the Battel of Asculum against the Romans in 279 BC, his losses were so great that he ultimately lost the war).

Success should not necessarily be equated with achieving the highest career position. In a very general sense, success can be defined as achieving a set objective. Therefore, success depends on the objectives that you set yourself.

But even this is not always quite clear.

Case Study 5
The High School Pupil Who Failed—And Nevertheless Succeeded
Years ago, a school pupil named Lea contacted me. During the course of working towards her abitur (general qualification for university entrance), she had compiled a questionnaire which she wanted to use to ask psychiatrists

questions about ADHD. It became apparent that the questions in the questionnaire did not fit the subfield that she was interested in. Answering them would have allowed no statements to be made about the hypothesis suggested by Lea.

I didn't answer the questions but rang her up to explain this to her. At first, Lea was totally desperate. She'd already received many completed forms and invested a great deal of time in data collection. The deadline for giving in her work was approaching. Her project was in danger of being a total failure.

But Lea nevertheless got top marks for her project.

She grasped that science does not deal with knowledge, but with ignorance. In other words: it's about transforming ignorance into new knowledge. That's exactly what she then implemented in her project. She explained her methodological errors with relentless clarity. Coherently she came to the conclusion that the formulation of the questions and the choice of method need to fit, and she explained needs to be considered in the process.

In terms of content, her project failed; but in terms of her scientific thinking, it was a major success. It represented a triumph of scientific integrity over prestige-oriented "fake" success.

Success in your job doesn't necessarily mean climbing to the highest position. Don't forget the Peter Principle (see Sect. 4.2.3): being promoted a step too high, meaning that you are out of your depth, is not only a catastrophe for your subordinates but above all for you yourself. It means an end to any kind of composure and joy at work but a total increase in overload and a fear of being found out.

Being successful means being in a place where you can—and also want—to use your abilities.

Case Study 6
The Woman Who Exercised Her Freedom
In the case of Miriam, a young woman whom I treated many years ago, it took me a long time until I understood that she was indeed successful.

The diagnosis ADHD was made as early as primary school with Miriam. For a while she was treated with medication with some success. However, her treatment cannot be interpreted as meaning that Miriam learned to understand her ADHD. She was simply taught that she could not do this or that.

Despite this, her school career was acceptable thanks to her exceptional intelligence, and she achieved a good secondary school leaving examination. Following this, she and a schoolfriend travelled through South America for a few months. When they returned, her friend began studying for a degree in mathematics.

Miriam herself found a job as a kind of receptionist in a large corporation. She sat there in the entrance lobby in a glass box.

- Her job was to tell visitors where they could find the offices of their contact partner.
- She also accepted personal deliveries for staff such as a pack of fresh laundry or food from the pizza courier, and then contact the respective employee.
- When times were busy, she helped out at the switchboard.

At the time she came to my practice, she had been doing this job for almost 10 years.

As I heard this story, in my arrogance I was horrified. It shouldn't be that this young intelligent woman was doing a job that lay way beneath her potential!

I explained my reasoning to Miriam very clearly.

She had already noticed that she wasn't stupid. It was just that whenever she had been given difficult tasks during her schooldays, she became anxious. A tumult of thoughts, solution approaches, possible sources of error and other things went through her head. Then she was plagued with great doubt as to whether she would be able to separate out all her thoughts. She suffered terribly from this. Even when she had been able to master this kind of task, the satisfaction did not last. Simply imagining the next task was horrendously stressful for her.

After graduating from high school, she said to herself that she had actually proved her intelligence and perseverance. She wanted decide about her own life herself, without having to conform to the requirements of anyone else or of society as a whole. So, she deliberately made the decision to follow a career which did not place any exceptional demands on her. She just wanted never again to have the feeling of being out of her depth. Her way of staying secure was the most important thing for her.

This status was the most important thing for her. The work she had chosen proved to be ideal for her. She was permanently in contact with the employees. In the meantime, she got to know many of them privately. She felt as if she was in a big family in this company where, despite being a young person, she had become a kind of surrogate mother or big sister.

In other words: Miriam had exercised the freedom not to overcome her fears owing to alleged overload in a more demanding job and have a big career. She gave herself the freedom to decide and thereby achieved a very high degree of satisfaction.

Strictly speaking, I first understood how Miriam had been successful in her life, after she had broken off her therapy with me. Even if I had understood Miriam's explanations cognitively, it was an effort for me to respect her position. In a roundabout way, I tried to persuade her to "make more" of her talents. She didn't appreciate this and broke off the therapy—rightly so.

I learned a lot about the essence of freedom and the essence of success from this encounter.

4.3   A Person Is Not Only ADHD

In the field of medicine, there is an expression in German which translates as "one can have lice and fleas at the same time". It reminds us doctors not to stop observing and thinking if we have found one cause for a symptom. A patient with itching could have fleas as well as lice, which also contribute to the itching.

In the context of the topic of ADHD and the world of work, I would simply like to point out that an ADHDer is not just ADHD. First and foremost an ADHDer is a person—somehow, more or less just like everyone else, even when one often feels "different" and even if there are actually certain differences. But we ADHDers are made up of more than just ADHD, even if ADHD can have an impact on all areas of our lives.

If you lose sight of this, it's easy to inadvertently define yourself only in terms of the ADHD and the "being different". This can rapidly happen, owing to the mere fact that a kind of wavelength often exists between ADHDers—a (mostly) pleasant mutual acknowledgement. Sometimes this is taken to such an extreme that the ADHD constitution is elevated, completely inappropriately, as being particularly desirable. In a worst-case scenario, the impression is created of belonging to an alleged elite.

This is of course ridiculous. ADHD is neither better nor worse than non-ADHD, in the same way that female is neither better nor worse than male.

Particularly in the world of work, however, it is extremely important to behave as a complete person, **with your complete identity**. This naturally also includes the ADHD-related characteristics and of course the weak spots as well. **To be successful, it's important not to allow yourself to be reduced to just ADHD, and not to define yourself solely through this perspective**.

And while we are on the topic of lice and fleas:

We humans can have psychological difficulties in life for all kinds of possible reasons such as relationship problems, addictive behaviour, fears, depressive moods, self-harm, eating disorders, authority problems and many more.

ADHD can lead to these kinds of difficulties. However even with ADHDers, these difficulties can have *other* causes.

It's necessary to differentiate between the following causal areas:

- Hereditary neurophysiological causes including the maldevelopment and misunderstandings that result from them (such as in ADHD or autism spectrum disorders).
- Reactive psychological difficulties such as feelings and experiences that the person has not yet worked though and which have therefore been shifted into the unconscious where they will be kept, wherever possible, using psychodynamic defence mechanisms. This is often combined with an unconscious urge to commit self-sabotage. These kinds of psychological difficulties used to be known as neuroses, a term which has disappeared from the official diagnosis codes but is still often used.

- Causes such as hormonal dysregulations, metabolic disorders, side effects of pharmaceuticals, poisonings and the like.
- Damage to the brain tissue through injury, deformity, long-standing alcohol consumption, etc.
- And also: naturally these areas can also appear simultaneously and influence each other.

All these areas can cause similar symptoms that can be easily mistaken for each other.

Examples:

- Impulsiveness can occur not only in ADHD but also in frontal lobe injuries such as after a brain injury. At the same time, these kinds of injuries can cause further symptoms which also occur in ADHD such as a lack of concentration and digressing from a topic.
- Motoric restlessness is one of the most common symptoms of ADHD. However, it also occurs in certain psychodynamic difficulties as a defence mechanism to non-specifically remove tension relating to the fear of one's own unresolved intense feelings.
- Provocative behaviour is quite common in ADHD. It occurs when an ADHDer impulsively comes out with an allegedly cool statement which is taken to be a provocation "by mistake". In contrast, the provocativeness in the case of psychodynamic difficulties occurs in the context of unconsciously intended self-sabotage (Lachenmeier 2013).

This list could be continued with countless other examples. In other words: a symptom, or even several symptoms together, does not yet say a great deal about the person affected. From the examples above, it is clear that the respective treatment must be different according to the underlying causes. So, if too much emphasis is placed on single symptom, a diagnostic and therapeutic misjudgement can be the result.

It's important that all those who consult medical psychiatric or psychological specialists about their difficulties are aware of this. Because unfortunately the fields of psychiatry and psychology currently focus too much on the level of a few symptoms and too little on the essence of being human and the essence of human suffering.

If you are uncertain or the situation is unclear, you should simply ask. In a friendly way, please, and not accusingly. Discuss your perceptions with the person treating you. Of course, some of the people treating you may not be used to this. As a young doctor I sometimes had to swallow hard in such situations, but I learned a lot in the process which I would otherwise have missed. But I hope that most of the specialists will ultimately be able to respond to your request.

If this is not possible after some effort on your part, then you may need to decide if you are being treated by the right specialist for you. Where possible, you should be given the opportunity to freely choose which physician or therapist will treat you.

It is important for patients to be able to decide who they choose to treat them. Ultimately, it's about your own life—or your own working life.

However, the reverse situation must also be accepted: it is right that physicians or psychologists can also decide themselves with whom they would like to work as patients.

References

Carlson GA, Kelly KL. Stimulant rebound: how common it is and what does it mean? J Child Adolesc Psychopharmacol. 2003;13:137–42.

Heller J. Something happened. New York: Alfred A. Knopf; 1974.

Lachenmeier H. Vortrag ADHS und ISTDP. Zurich; 2013. https://istdp.ch/sites/default/files/downloadfiles/HeiLac_ADHSuISTDP.pdf.

Peter LJ, Hull R. The Peter principle. New York: William Morrow; 1969.

Riedel A. Klinische Diagnostik und Erfahrungen aus der Sprechstunde für Autismus-Spektrum-Störungen. In: Tebartz van Elst l (pub.). Das Asperger-Syndrom im Erwachsenenalter. Berlin: Medizinisch Wissenschaftliche Verlagsgesellschaft; 2013.

Schlösser C. ADHS im Erwachsenenalter. Aktuell Psychiatr Psychother. 2006;6:12–4.

Weiss L. A.D.D. on the Job. Dallas: Taylor Publishing Company; 1996.

Directly Job-Related: ADHD Works!

5

In this chapter, I will illustrate a selection of important aspects and mechanisms of ADHD and their potential influence on working life, and demonstrate some options for a constructive coping strategy.

5.1   Starting a New Job: The Special ADHD Learning Curve

I have experienced several times that a professionally successful ADHDer with a great deal of experience is fired during the probationary period after changing to another company. And they were intelligent, capable professionals who had long mastered the tasks required of them—both technically and also in terms of their personality. Despite this, they were unable to cope, couldn't understand what had happened and ended up with huge self-doubt and resignation, even as far as depression.

Case Study 7: Part One

The Successful Businesswoman Who Crashed when the Job Conditions Were Perfect, and Was Only Resurrected Years Later

Sabine grew up in a small community in the country. Her father was a craftsman; her mother was a housewife. As a child she spent a lot of time daydreaming, often appeared to be absent and did not show much interest in school. Nobody was expecting much of her. In her village she was known and loved as a nice girl. She just managed to get through her time at school. An aunt helped her get an apprenticeship at the local town hall. She felt at home in the familiar environment of the small village and passed her apprenticeship after three years' training.

© The Author(s), under exclusive license to Springer Nature Switzerland AG 2023
H. Lachenmeier, *ADHD and Success at Work*,
https://doi.org/10.1007/978-3-031-13437-1_5

At that time, a friend of the family began to set up a backyard business. He asked Sabine if she could do the paperwork for him. So, she changed from the trusted town hall to the small new business of her trusted neighbour. She organised the office, which was still small. The backyard business grew in time. Step-by-step Sabine developed the administrative areas. Further tasks were added such as work contracts with mechanics, salespeople and administrative employees; payroll accounting, budget planning and much more. The small garage grew into a large car dealership with around 20 employees.

Step-by-step Sabine developed to become the skilled, respected boss of commercial and administrative affairs. She was rightly proud of her career path.

The owner was satisfied with her in every way and had continually raised her salary. At some point, he said that he wanted nothing more than for her to continue to work for him. But he could understand if, with her quality and experience, she aspired to more lofty professional goals. He would not stand in her way, although he would be very sorry to lose her. On the contrary, he would be thankful. He would also finance advanced training for her, if she wanted to do it.

After careful consideration, Sabine applied for a similarly challenging job in a designer furniture shop in Zurich. She got the job, against several competitors, thanks to her experience and qualifications.

Full of zeal, she started the new job. After just a few days, she was completely bewildered because she just didn't seem able to cope. The processes were not the same as the ones she was used to. She didn't know the people yet, nor the company culture. Attempting to get everything done nevertheless, with great expenditure of time, she made several serious mistakes. Because of this, she did not live up to the expectations of her employer, nor of course to her own expectations either. She was already fired during the probationary period.

After this experience, she was completely confused. She had never made mistakes like these in all the years working for the other company. After her schooldays and apprenticeship, she had only been successful.

And now this. But Sabine pulled herself together, looked for a new job— and experienced the same thing again. Even when she took on jobs that were less challenging, the same thing happened. She became unemployed. Her morale sank. Her marriage experienced a crisis and eventually she got divorced. Sabine was confused.

Ultimately she was admitted to hospital with the diagnosis of depression. Various drug and non-drug treatments brought no lasting success. She suffered relapses, was re-admitted to hospital, was considered for a disability pension. Finally, during her last stay in hospital she received her diagnosis from a young doctor who also had ADHD.

5.1.1   Important to Know: An Advantage in the Long-Term but Limiting in the Short-Term

In order to understand the story of Sabine described above, we need to consider the type of learning and/or the way information is absorbed. And in the wider sense, how the process of getting to know a specialist field, an organisation or a company takes place. This includes countless banal snippets of information about the context such as where do I find the paper for the printer or who has had conflict or whatever with whom.

> **Encore**
> The differences between non-ADHD and ADHD as they are explained below correspond to the fundamental way that the two groups function, i.e. a kind of original state.
> Of course, every ADHDer develops numerous different coping mechanisms. These can also include the ones that allow you to get an overview at a new location particularly quickly.

Through the automatic weighting of the information that bombards them, **non-ADHDers** are able to separate the important information from the unimportant. They rapidly receive an initial overview, distinguish the "motorways" from the "side streets" so to speak, get their bearings quickly and can soon reliably deal with the most important routine tasks. Their learning curve rises correspondingly quickly at the beginning. Then the curve flattens out – through experience, one or two things are added and finally a plateau is reached.

ADHDers do not have this filter—or they have it to a lesser extent—so they try to take "everything" on board, no matter whether it's important or not. In other words, everything that happens to appear under their nose. Naturally this is not possible. What sticks at the beginning is a partly random selection.

Thereby, initially, some of the most important and simplest things are missed. The randomly absorbed selection of information remains incoherent—at first. You have the impression that you don't understand anything and doubt your abilities. The learning curve bobs up and down at around the zero line, or so it seems.

If you manage to hold on for long enough, then you will gradually acquire detailed information across the entire subject area. At some point you will also get an overall view, but with a far greater level of detail. All the isolated information will fit together like a puzzle. When this happens, "everything" will become clear to you, from one day to the next. The learning curve rises almost vertically, and it normally rises higher than that of a non-ADHDer of the same intelligence (Fig. 5.1).

The reason for this is that not only do you get an overview, you absorb a tremendous number of details at the same time. You have thus not only explored the

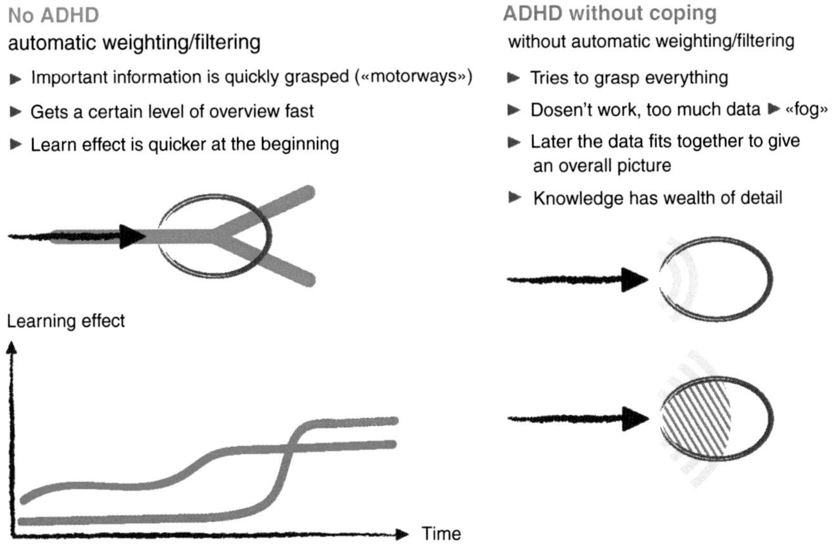

No ADHD
automatic weighting/filtering

▶ Important information is quickly grasped («motorways»)

▶ Gets a certain level of overview fast

▶ Learn effect is quicker at the beginning

ADHD without coping
without automatic weighting/filtering

▶ Tries to grasp everything

▶ Dosen't work, too much data ▶ «fog»

▶ Later the data fits together to give
  an overall picture

▶ Knowledge has wealth of detail

Learning effect

Time

Fig. 5.1 Different learning curves in ADHD and non-ADHD

"motorways and main roads", but also the side streets and farm tracks, and you know who lives in the small alleyway next to the market square on the third floor. Intelligent ADHDers are therefore particularly quick thinking in the areas in which they have concentrated their full interest, and particularly able to discover and deploy correlations and solution possibilities.

If you have just identified this plausible pattern, it is amazing how often these kinds of learning curve can be found in the life stories of ADHDers.

With these realisations, it's easy to understand why the ADHDers mentioned at the beginning unexpectedly failed after changing their job. None of them knew anything about the unequal mechanisms when learning—about the different learning curve.

They were not aware of the extent of their knowledge in their former job, both technically and contextually. And how much security this had given them. They were all understandably shocked that, despite their specialist knowledge, they had difficulty in getting to grips with their new location. They stumbled almost blindly into a "data tsunami".

This is what usually happens:

• During the first, flat phase, you get the impression that you have not absorbed any information; although you have actually saved numerous facts, they do not yet fit together sufficiently to make the picture complete.

• The fact that you hardly feel any learning success leads you inevitably to doubt your own value.

• This is increasingly followed by the fear of not being good enough and of being exposed by superiors and colleagues as being not good enough.

• The fear also distracts you, and you make mistakes or errors. You try to either cover these up or you apologise excessively.

- Your superiors gradually become aware of this. They also begin to have doubts about their new employee.
- A vicious circle increasingly develops which can easily end in disaster.

It certainly doesn't have to be like this.

Case Study 7: Part Two

The Successful Businesswoman Who Crashed When the Job Conditions Were Perfect, and Was Only Resurrected Years Later

The young hospital doctor who had made the diagnosis started to teach Sabine about ADHD and its influence on her life. Her previous high-dose treatment with anti-depressive drugs was reduced and combined with stimulants (methylphenidate). Sabine soon felt better.

Sabine was referred to my practice for her continuing outpatient treatment. Over a period lasting several months, we talked about the way in which ADHD functioned and compared it with numerous situations in her life.

She began to understand how she had enjoyed no insecurities whatsoever in the familiar environment of her village and the car dealership—jobs which developed step by step. She knew everything and everyone inside out and always had a complete overview. Not only from a general perspective, but in every detail. However, she was not conscious of this.

Without realising about her ADHD and its laws of function, and with her history, Sabine had almost no chance when she started at the same occupational level in an unfamiliar environment. She did not know about the different learning curve. Understandably, the new experience of professional uncertainty made her feel insecure; she was plagued with despair, self-doubt and finally resignation and depressive moods. This range of symptoms can be easily confused with clinical depression if symptoms and phenomenological findings are not ascertained precisely enough (Neuhaus 2005).

When she was able to understand these processes, Sabine could recognise that the fact that she came to grief in the furniture shop had nothing to do with her lack of ability. She understood how it happened. Even more important: knowing how ADHD functions in this way, she learned how to retain the medium-term advantage and how to specifically minimise the short-term disadvantage, and sometimes even completely prevent it.

And last but not least: she recognised again, and not only cognitively but also emotionally; how great her potential is. She gained courage; dared to do things that she would have never dared to do earlier (see also Sect. 7.1).

Subsequently she decided to take entrance test to train as an educator for adults at the age of 47. She not only passed the entrance test but successfully completed the training. Later she completed a thorough advanced training course in coaching. Sabine has now been working very successfully again for 15 years. Today she has a managerial post in a prestigious agency for executive coaching in Zurich.

Truly a phoenix risen from the ashes.

5.1.2   Suggested Solutions When Changing Jobs

The fundamentals of almost every sensible coping mechanism with ADHD are:

- To make sure you get an orientation and overview manually, because you are less able to automatically distinguish what information is important.
- To consciously monitor and regulate yourself, because the control centre of your executive functions is less active.
- To keep an eye on the fact that if you have difficulties, you shouldn't doubt your self-worth in a knee-jerk reaction, but assess yourself in the context of reality.

Naturally this isn't always easy. Sometimes absolutely banal things that are easy to implement can be helpful here. And you can use your knowledge about the way in which ADHD functions.

5.1.2.1 Before Changing Jobs

It's a good idea to find out in advance about a few banal conditions at your new place of work. These can help to give you orientation points when you are flooded with data during the first few days. Firstly, you will reduce the uncertainty (fear) of the first day at work and secondly, the orientation points will serve as a structure to help you classify and save the large amount of new information.

These banal conditions often prove to be astonishingly effective orientation points.

> **Encore**
> ADHDer who are rather intelligent often regard these tricks as being somehow beneath them. But they can profit from them in particular: the more intelligent you are, the more associations you produce for every new input. And therefore the faster you lose sight of the big picture. The insecurity that results from this as an emotional reaction to the banal things that happen on the first day at work in a company can affect you with an unexpected intensity.
>
> In brief: it is smart to prepare yourself as an ADHDer for the possible negative consequences ($\approx$ side effects) of your own cleverness.

The following techniques have proved useful:

- Find out about your route to work in advance.
- Find out about the surrounding area in advance: the building, canteen, smoking area, toilets, relaxation or quiet rooms, shopping possibilities, park, etc.
- Print out an organigram of the future company or new department; possibly add the names and even photos of a few (!) people who you need to know.
- Convert the job description into a brief overview diagram, and only roughly outline it: because "if I undertake to produce a perfect overview diagram, I will never finish it anyway".
- etc.

5.1.2.2 Starting in a New Place: Dealing with Yourself

If you are aware of the reason why your learning curve can be slow at the beginning, you are not surprised if it happens. You don't fall into a panic or get stressed so quickly. Instead, you are able to trust that with enough time, everything will come together and you will be able to fulfil the requirements of the appropriately chosen job.

> **Encore**
>
> It can be helpful to look for an example that illustrates this learning curve from your own life and where you have learned that ultimately you were able to master it particularly successfully. Logically we tend to trust a model which arises from our own experience most of all. It is able to resist any possible increasing pressure most effectively.

The knowledge about the difference between ADHD and non-ADHD can also be used to speed up your own learning curve.

The ADHD condition definitely does not mean an inability to prioritise and to filter, but merely that less automatic pre-filtering takes place. If I am aware of this, then I can consciously—i.e. manually—decide what is important and make a note of it, from the first day onwards.

- It's important not to simply rely on your memory, even if it is otherwise good. You will save a lot of effort if you simply make a note of everything right from the beginning. Absolutely everything—even things that you are sure you will never forget! It doesn't matter whether you do this in a notebook or on your mobile phone; the important thing is to do it immediately, in the moment.
- For the first few weeks, it's a good idea to filter out the day's three most important pieces of information every evening, to underline them and make a mental note of them. Take three to four minutes maximum for this task. This is easily long enough and one is hardly able to cope with more, anyway.
- To increase your perception of self-worth: every evening, make a note of three positive aspects of your working day. Plus one which you would like to improve on.

In this way, you can combine the non-ADHD advantages with learning about ADHD, and you will be able to have your cake and eat it, or as the Swiss say, take your "Weggli" (bread roll) and keep the five "Rappen!" (pennies).

5.1.2.3 Starting in a New Place: Dealing with Your Superiors and Colleagues

As mentioned above, superiors and managers can also become nervous in this first phase if they notice that their new employee is not (yet) getting off the ground. This is understandable. But if I now know how things work with me as an ADHDer, I can sense enough self-confidence to speak about it with my superiors pre-emptively.

If you speak to your superior, bear the following in mind:

- The label "ADHD" is not the primary point of focus (see Sect. 4.1).
- It's not at all about demanding pity or being given special treatment across the board.
- The aim is much more to make the superior worry less that he has made the wrong decision in selecting you and that he cannot rely on you.
- And that the superior continues to see your fundamental competence and commitment, and therefore can be confident in giving you a little more time to adjust.

It is also a good idea—usually without mentioning the term ADHD—to give a simple, clear but positive message such as for example:

It's important to me that I do the tasks completely correctly here. I don't want to hurry through anything and do it wrong. That's why I am a little bit more hesitant than others at the beginning and need a little more time until I have got a secure overview. But as soon as I have familiarised myself with the tasks, you will be able to rely on me completely.

Naturally this procedure is only justified if it actually corresponds to the situation and your abilities. In other words: when the trust that you would like to have is justified.

5.1.2.4 A Banal but Important Distinction

In the initial situation, when you are flooded with information, impressions and thoughts, a banal difference can help you to get your bearings better. The induction period in a new job can be mentally divided into two areas:

- Specialist and organisational induction
- Induction in terms of relationships and communication

Often our feelings of disorientation lead us to focus too much on the specialist side of the induction.

We pay less attention to the second part. But this part is even more important for ADHDers in several ways. It is not only related to possible communication about the learning curve. In ADHDers, it's easy for banal, communicative obvious skills which one would normally be familiar with to get lost.

For example, an IT specialist who had started a new job in IT for a university research institution, had simply not thought about giving a short acknowledgement of receipt and rough time estimation of completion for the questions and commissions he was receiving from the scientists. He left them in the dark, so to speak, meaning that his personal integration at the new location was more difficult than necessary. This would not have happened to him if, during the induction phase, he had consciously and repeatedly visualised the differentiation: specialist/organisational and relationship/communication.

5.2   ADHD and Chronic Stress: Burnout

Now I'm going to make myself unpopular for a moment:

- Life *is* strenuous. There's no getting away from it—it's normal.
- Not everyone who is in a burnout has achieved a great deal.

However: burnout (Burisch 1989), also defined as extreme emotional and physical exhaustion, causes a great deal of suffering. It is more prevalent in ADHDers. There are reasons for this and if you know about it, you can at least partly do something about it.

> **Encore**
> Stress can be defined as feeling burdened or tense. Hans Selye who first coined the term stress (Selye 1936) describes eustress as the "salt of life", without which life would be boring. As with salt, too much is not good (distress), but not enough is also not good. Both lead to a similar condition, known as burnout in one case and "boreout" in the other.

Stress can be damaging primarily when the burden is excessive on a long-term basis (chronic). This is dependent on:

- Quantity of work, but not only this.
- Emotional burdens through the type of work such as nursing, criminal investigation by the police, psychotherapy and others.
- Personal, emotionally straining relationships at work such as a derogatory atmosphere; managerial weakness; contradictory, so-called double-bind (dilemma) communication from superiors; but also, hostile attitude from inferiors towards their superiors; intrigues, including from below to the top; etc.
- How someone reacts to the work situation and burdens, although increased insecurity and fear are the decisive factors.
- And never forget: to honestly consider whether the stress is based on the fact that you do not have the specialist abilities or experience required for the tasks.

How does ADHD have an effect on this? How come there is increased energy consumption with ADHD?—As always in such considerations, it's worth taking a look at the fundamental functional patterns: the filter and control models.

5.2.1   Overload Owing to Unchecked Thinking

In ADHD, the information that comes into your brain from outside, the individual memory content that is mobilised and the thoughts and associations that are triggered are separated to a lesser extent into important and less important.

The first consequence of this is both banal and serious: the brain of an ADHDer has to process much more information—and not only for short moments of time, but permanently.

This can easily lead to a quantitative-cognitive overload, because brains are like computers: the more data that have to be processed, the more energy is used.

Encore
Even though this direct overload caused by unchecked thinking is impressive in terms of mere volume, it does not play the main role in the development of exhaustion conditions in ADHD.

The weight of our brain makes up around 2% of our body but the brain uses 20–30% of the entire energy needs of a person, depending on the situation (Lennie 2003). Pure thinking however does not require that much energy. The really big energy consumers in our brain are feelings, above all burdensome feelings such as insecurity, fear, self-doubt and feelings of guilt. But positive feelings also consume a lot of energy.

And of course, the "pure thinking" mentioned above is rather rare. Associated feelings are usually involved in the thinking. It's clear to everyone that when making the decision to expand a company and employ another member of staff, not only cold figures play a role but also the uncertainty or fear of the risk associated with this.

5.2.2   Uncertainty in the Flood of Data: "Fog of Anxiety"

The second consequence of the reduced filtering lies in the difficulty of gaining an overview in the midst of a surplus of information and thoughts. The numerous, initially incoherent data produce a chaotic clutter, a "data fog".

The fact that you don't at first have an overview in the data fog therefore logically triggers a feeling of uncertainty. This uncertainty is caused by a lack of orientation in the fog and can best be described as a "fog of anxiety" (Fig. 5.2).

This chronically repetitive uncertainty, which is created by the permanent flood of data, is a severe devourer of energy and can be stronger or weaker, depending on the situation. It can contribute decisively to the development of exhaustion.

Naturally within the turmoil created by this uncertainty, there is also the potential to discover or invent new things, through your thinking and associations. This can be a very sought-after skill in certain special situations, but can occasionally be awkward in normal everyday working life.

The fog of anxiety described often triggers torturous self-doubt. It impedes the perception of one's self-worth. Ultimately, one becomes less willing to achieve good performance and reduces one's ambitions. Or one reacts in a compensatory way by being even more ambitious, and is only satisfied when one is "perfect".

Careful: even ADHDers who appear to be very self-assured on the outside and are professionally very successful often suffer from these self-doubts! They usually

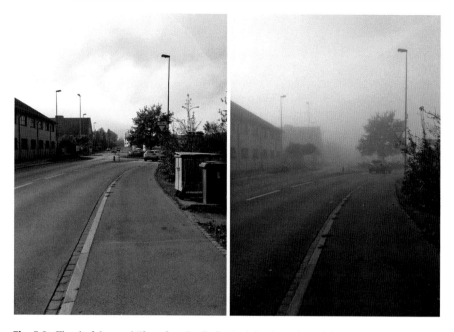

Fig. 5.2 Flood of data and "fog of anxiety". On the left, clear view without ADHD. On the right with ADHD → too much data → uncertainty/anxiety like in fog

hide these doubts, though, because they themselves cannot understand what continues to drive their self-doubt. This vicious circle is easiest to break if the ADHD-functional processes that led to it can be understood precisely on an individual basis.

A further devastating consequence of the "fog of anxiety" that is often seen is an inability to decide which task really belongs to me, or whether a third party is wrongly trying to push something on to me and whether I am entitled to defend myself or not, and so on.

As a consequence of this, ADHDers often have problems with setting boundaries, with saying no and along with this, to assert or defend themselves.

Encore
Important: these problems often appear to be confusingly similar to the consequences of unresolved unconscious feelings and conflicts, in other words from psychodynamic difficulties (formerly known as: neurotic difficulties). When they have developed because of ADHD processes, as described above, they are very much easier for the person affected to solve.

Conversely, the following also applies: therapy that focusses on unconscious conflicts would be of no use if the person exhibits inhibition that is caused by ADHD fog of anxiety. It would be much more likely to cause confusion and tend to lead to even more uncertainty.

5.2.3   Coping and Its Possible Stress Side Effects

Target-oriented coping mechanisms can also have side effects. An astonishing number of ADHDers use the fundamental coping strategy of overcompensating.

There is a series of fundamental coping strategies that often form contrasting pairs. I will explain two of them in relation to chronic stress:

5.2.3.1 Contrasting Pair: "Overcompensating" Versus "Intuitive-Figurative Pattern"

A first contrasting pair is when a person tends to either think through and check through something point for point, and in this sense overcompensates; or tends to perceive things in an intuitive-figurative way and perceive the "big picture".

These kinds of contrasting pairs often occur in the same person simultaneously where they are used as coping mechanisms.

Case Study 8
The Management Consultant Who Stayed Right on Course in the Fog, but Didn't Realise It

Naturally, these contrasting pairs can also exist simultaneously in the same individual. I recall the case of the management consultant Talula, aged between 50 and 60 with two adult children.

Talula is an exceptionally experienced adviser, sharp as a nail, well-known for her clear approach, sensitive and understanding and nevertheless ready for hard confrontation wherever it is necessary. She can hold her position unwaveringly, if she firmly believes in it. She is nevertheless open at any time for legitimate objections; those that are unsubstantiated make her hit the roof immediately.

Tabula is a perfectionist in technical matters: she follows up every improbable branch line, without losing sight of where the journey is going. She is prepared to undertake additional research in her free time or complete the documentation of work for her clients. It's hardly surprising that she was awarded an advancement award when she was still at university.

In this respect, Talula demonstrates the typical image of a talented ADHDer with the fundamental coping strategy of overcompensating, and occasional impulsiveness. Successful in her job, with a great deal of knowledge and experience in her field.

She gained her sense of certainty mainly from overcompensating, her broad wealth of experience and knowledge in her field.

Owing to an unhappy chain of different circumstances, she ended up in a situation in which she had to represent the interests of a company for whom she occasionally worked, at a political level. It was a matter of existential importance for the company and lasted for several months.

Political work in the narrow sense was something which Talula had never come across; nor was it a field that had ever interested her. Naturally it was intellectually clear to her that the people involved in politics were no different to those in business life. However, she did not have any experience regarding

---

insider knowledge about the practices, the dos and don'ts in the subculture of politics. Naturally she was aware of the most relevant political parties, but was not familiar with their entanglements, the political minefield and the other problems buried all over the place.

In this situation, Talula experienced a feeling of insecurity which she had not felt in her job for decades, a fear that she remembered from when she was younger. Old insecurities came to the surface. She was tormented by a feeling of disorientation.

Subliminally however, Talula recognised the pattern and structures in this new field. She even imperceptibly absorbed the characteristics of the different stakeholders. But cognitively she was unsure about all these perceptions, had doubts and felt as if she was travelling in the fog without a compass. The stress was enormous.

It subsequently became clear to her:

Despite the conscious, intellectual insecurity, despite the emotionally impression of not being able to rely on her impressions, Talula had orientated herself on the subliminal perception of the pattern. However, she had done this without being aware of it and without feeling it.

She was affected by enormous stress: a fear that almost made her give up. Contrary to her subjective perception, however, she had followed the correct procedure "to-the-letter". After Talula had recognised her ADHD-functional processes, she could begin to recognise the potency of her decision made on the basis of intuitive-figurative perception—and to trust it.

She continued to gain security from overcompensating where necessary, but also additionally from her subliminal intuitive-figurative perception of patterns, which functioned very reliably in her case.

P.S. In order to avoid misunderstandings: the reliability of this intuitive-figurative assessment is naturally not absolute. In particular if someone has fallen into negative hyperfocus (tunnel vision), then they cannot rely on it at all (see also Sect. 6.4).

5.2.3.2 Contrasting Pair: "Overcompensating" Versus "Doing Nothing"

Together with another mechanism, the coping strategy of overcompensating forms an even more extreme contrasting pair:

With this contrasting pair, when the person has new a task or a new area that has to be explored, either *generally nothing* is done (the thought tree is blocked before it starts), which leads to chaos, and usually makes any kind of success impossible.

Or the person does *generally everything*, regarding this to be a completely normal state of affairs; whenever you try to get something done, it's always like this. You therefore strive for perfectionism. In the process you learn a great deal, get a lot done, have success but at the price of very high energy consumption and the price that usually you have neither time nor energy for anything apart from your work. As a result, your private life (relationships, hobbies etc.) suffers.

It's quite often to meet ADHDers who are scrupulously exacting in their job but live in a messy apartment. And vice versa (Fig. 5.3).

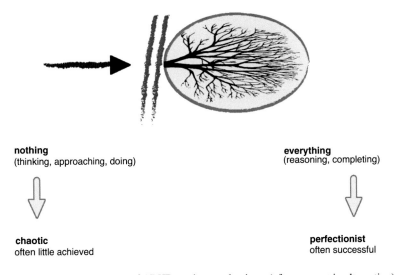

nothing
(thinking, approaching, doing)

everything
(reasoning, completing)

chaotic
often little achieved

perfectionist
often successful

Fig. 5.3 Two extreme variations of ADHD coping mechanisms (often present in alternation): all or nothing

The irony of this contrasting pair is that both actually *have the same purpose:* namely, not making a decision about what is important and what is not. It's just that one person achieves this by generally doing nothing. And the other achieves this by generally doing everything, meaning that they don't have to make a decision about what they leave out.

Both variations result in a raised chronic stress level.

Naturally this "all" or "nothing" approach should not be taken literally. Doing absolutely nothing would literally lead to death. Doing absolutely everything is impossible: no person can be really perfect.

5.2.4   More ADHD-Typical Behaviour That Can Wear You Down

Other typical ADHD processes can lead to increased stress and exhaustion to a considerable extent. I mention only a few of them here, such as the easily triggered negative hyperfocus. This leads to incorrect self-assessments and assessments about you from others, which create inter-personal tensions at work. ADHDers are more likely to put their foot in it, whether it's through reduced impulse control or because the overall context of a situation is not perceived for a moment. Impulsive interrupting is rarely appreciated. A lack of distance can, in its discreet manifestation, contribute to the charm of ADHDers, but it exceeds the accepted level very quickly in a professional context.

All this together can lead to painstakingly difficult work relationships that are filled with misunderstandings and massively increase your stress level.

5.2.5   Suggested Solutions for Chronic Stress

Very different strategies can be required depending on the personal situation, which must all be individually processed. Here are some selected tips that make sense in most of the constellations. Fundamentally it's about gaining an overview and orientation here—as always in ADHD.

5.2.5.1 Job Description and List of Duties

As banal as it sounds: it's worth reading through your work contract, your job description and the accompanying list of duties.

With many ADHDers, a veil of "cannot-exactly-remember-anymore" can develop over time. Unnoticed, the boundaries to the duties that were assigned to you can become blurred. In this uncertainty—paired with chronic latent self-doubt—it is easy for the boundaries of these tasks to become much too wide "to be on the safe side". This leads to you becoming overburdened and possibly also to wrangling about responsibilities.

With a little bit of luck, repeating this check once in a while could not only rein in the burden of work, but above all, help you feel more secure and better equipped for your tasks. Both reduce stress.

5.2.5.2 Using a Routine to Stop Thinking

Unchecked ADHD thinking depletes your energy. Naturally one cannot just "not think", even if some ADHDers often wish that they could do just that (it's not that ADHDers think too little—they just think too widely). It's also natural not to want to stop thinking entirely because this superb human idiosyncrasy is so important for ADHDers.

But: in certain cases, it's possible to ensure that you don't even begin to do—unproductive—thinking. In this way, you can achieve "non-thinking" in a very smart way!

Among the duties that periodically occur in the world of work and private life, there are many boring, laborious and recurring tasks. These are often postponed under the motto "should I start today, or first tomorrow and why didn't I start yesterday?" This approach uses an enormous amount of energy, above all through the third part: a combination of guilty conscience including self-reproach (Fig. 5.4).

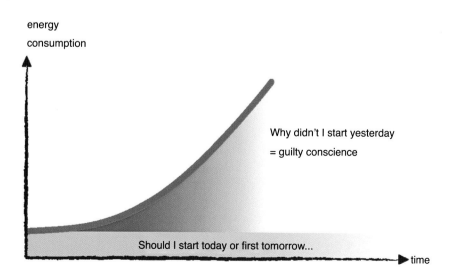

Fig. 5.4   "Should I start today, or first tomorrow, and why didn't I start yesterday?"

Encore

Of course, in the case of such boring recurrent work there is, as is so often the case with ADHD, also a diametrically opposite coping method. Some people even enjoy doing these kinds of tasks, using their filing or housework chores as an opportunity not to have to think about anything and thereby to be able to escape their driven inner restlessness for a moment and relax.

For these kinds of recurrent boring/tedious duties, it's hardly worth starting with deliberations such as "should I start today, or first tomorrow, and why didn't I start yesterday?" Owing to your unchecked thinking, you'll never come to a stop as there are so many possible variations to consider. In order to avoid the complete weighing up and decision-making procedure here, the tendency is then to postpone carrying out these tasks.

If you really decide internally to do them (without making an internal genuine decision on your part it doesn't work—an "attempt" or "intent" is not sufficient), it's a good idea to establish a rhythm for these tasks.

- This could be a defined time during which you regularly deal with complaint emails, for example, do the filing or clear your workspace.
- Functional instead of time guidelines are also useful. For example, I write health insurance reports when the pile of requests has reached the 10 cm level and not one millimetre later—but also not earlier than then.

The point of having a fixed rhythm or routine is that you then do not need to think about it. Pondering about something and making a decision become obsolete.

You are now going to say to me that this is easier said than done. Of course! It requires a certain amount of effort to decide on a rhythm and also to keep to it. However, this is a one-off decision. You don't have to make a new decision every single time you have a recurrent task to do.

It's a good idea to begin gently with one single area of your life, and give yourself enough time to get used to it.

And if you feel like protesting that structures are restricting, then I would have agreed with you when I was younger. At that time, I hadn't understood that useful structures can expand your level of freedom and actually not restrict it. Useful structures save my time and energy for the things that are important to me.

Important: The following points are decisive, if a routine is to be successful:

- It only works if you have made an internal decision for yourself, and cannot be imposed from outside. If you try to order yourself to do something, it doesn't work either.
- It's also important to specify how often the rhythm may be broken during a defined period, because:

We ADHDers absolutely need rules and structures—but we don't need to slavishly follow them *all the time.*
For example:
Rhythm for doing the filing: Monday and Thursday: 15.00–16.00
Duration period: 1 month
Flexibility: skip it two times maximum

- Decide what you want to do if you have a "permitted" interruption of the rhythm, so that you don't start thinking like crazy again.

  In the example above, this means that if I skip the rhythm of the routine once, then I don't try to "catch up" in between, because: the next rhythmic beat is close enough—my routine remains within acceptable limits.

- If the flexibility options are not used up during one period of time, they may *not* be transferred to the next period. Experience has shown that otherwise, almost everyone then starts to collect flexibility points. At some point, this results in a longer break in the routine, as a result of which the self-chosen rhythm is lost, and with it the relieving effect.

Encore
On the topic of "constructive thinking stop and rhythm" it is also important to clearly divide up time periods. "Working from... to..." and perhaps more importantly "not working from... to...". This applies to breaks during work, but also, for example, to the definition of the latest possible time you can stop work for the day.

- In this way, you will be able to keep going more easily during the working phase, because the end of the day is clearly defined and "within sight".
- At the same time, you will find the work breaks more refreshing because the fact that they are clearly defined means that you should not be disturbed by thoughts such as "shouldn't I continue working?" Your breaks are secure, reserved time pockets and clear orientation points.

5.2.5.3 General Orientation in Situations

As you are now aware, in ADHD "pre-filtering" of information and thoughts takes place less automatically. This means that ADHDers are required to get their initial overview or orientation themselves—manually, so to speak.

Encore
Warning: people often misunderstand the term filter: it's about filtering, not about censoring. With a filter, important information is included and unimportant information is left out (but not forbidden). If it were censorship, most of the important information would be forbidden and a lot of unimportant or even false information would be communicated.

With a few sensible criteria which you can focus on, it's possible to find your orientation in an unclear situation. In the same way that people divide a three-dimensional space with the help of three axis, it can be helpful to assess new situations according to the three criteria listed below. In almost every professional (or private) situation, it's possible to get an initial overview, a first orientation in a useful period of time with this method.

- *Order of Magnitude*
  - Important/unimportant or expensive/cheap or affects many people/affects individuals or global significance/local significance, etc.
- *Perspective*
  - My point of view/point of view of the other person or my personal-private point of view/my point of view as a professional or today's point of view/ point of view in a year or look into the future/look back to the past, etc.
- *Jurisdiction/Responsibility*
  - Which part of a situation is my responsibility; which is not; and if so, who is responsible for it.

If it is a something small (order of magnitude) that will no longer play a role in a week (perspective), and is also under the management of my colleague (jurisdiction/responsibility), I can ignore the whole thing.

But I am free, as a friend of the person concerned, to decide on my part (my responsibility) to point out to him what he has overlooked. It is his responsibility whether he accepts this hint or not.

- ADHDers are at risk of initially perceiving facts as being too important. They can often prevent this by briefly checking the order of magnitude.
- At the same time, there is a danger of long-term consequences if something relevant, which is initially perceived as being boring, is ignored and not taken seriously enough. This risk can be eliminated by checking the perspective.
- If you do not get a clear picture when assigning responsibilities, your unsolicited work or efforts to help can easily be perceived by colleagues as interfering. The result is wrangling over competences, entanglements and disasters, in keeping with the motto: "the opposite of good is not bad, but well-intentioned".

5.2.5.4 Overview of the Relevance of the Tasks to Be Completed

I would now like to address a delicate topic, which I deliberate didn't attach to the above considerations on "Job description and list of duties". I don't want you to get the impression that I am suggesting you should not perform your duties correctly. This is definitely not the case. On the contrary. And this is despite the fact that I advise many ADHDers (although not all!) to work *less*. But usually in order to achieve *more*. But also to have more space for the more creative areas of your work, and to hopefully save some energy for your private life.

Encore

The idea of working less to achieve more may sound a little like "pie in the sky". It is not a promise but a hint on how one could *possibly but tangibly* achieve something in this direction. Not to lose yourself so often in detours. Sometimes this works better, sometimes less.

Or to put it briefly:

Perfectionism makes perfect sense in only a few cases. Otherwise, striving for perfectionism sometimes prevents everything.

The basic idea is quite simple and starts from the observations about coping with overcompensating owing to a tendency towards perfectionism. The urge to do simply everything and to do it as perfectly as possible, so as not to have to weigh up and decide anything in the flood of data. It is actually too time-consuming if, for each individual task, it is always necessary to weigh up time and again exactly what to do or not to do, and to find out in each individual detail what varying degrees of perfection are expected of me in carrying out the task. Without thinking, simply getting everything done seems less stressful.

The following method has proved to be successful. It's banal, but smart: create a simple grid which you can use to divide all your tasks into a few categories. Without thinking about everything from scratch every time. Once you have defined this grid, the categorisation becomes quite easy over time.

I suggest you use three categories for the grid:

- *Zero Tolerance*
    - These are tasks that must be absolutely fully completed without exception in a useful period of time such as "submitting the tax return of your own business", "showing up for an interview on time", "providing the figures for the balance sheet", "stopping arterial bleeding now", "activating the alarm system when closing the jewellery store", etc.

    Fortunately, these make up only a small proportion of the total number of possible tasks one may be faced will.
- *80/80*
    - This refers to tasks for which it is sufficient if 80% are completed on time with a degree of completeness or perfection of 80%. This is roughly the completion rate with which you would be in the "midfield" compared to other employees at the same level.

    You may be wondering how much does 80% mean. Well: it's a lot, but much less than what you *think* you should do.

    According to general experience, the 80/80 category is likely to represent the majority of professional tasks *required*—even in top managerial positions.
- *Nice to Have*
    - With these tasks, it is good when they are done. You may even like doing some of them. But they are unimportant; at a pinch they can also be omitted altogether.

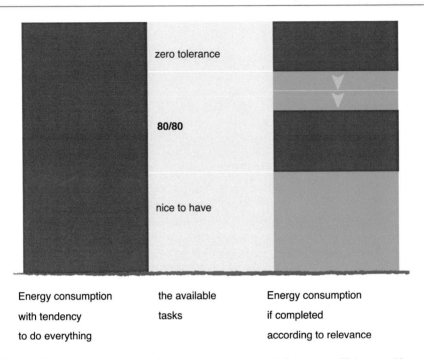

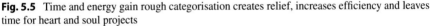

Energy consumption	the available	Energy consumption
with tendency	tasks	if completed
to do everything		according to relevance

Fig. 5.5 Time and energy gain rough categorisation creates relief, increases efficiency and leaves time for heart and soul projects

ADHDers usually do not spontaneously recognise these tasks as "irrelevant" or "not required". Especially when it comes to tasks that they particularly like to do. "nice to have" can also include wanting to complete a task that could be done well enough at "80/80" level nevertheless at "zero tolerance" level!

The category "nice to have" usually accounts for an astonishingly large proportion of one's—presumed—duties.

Shown schematically, the following illustration shows the great time-saving and energy-saving potential of this categorisation. You can even save time and energy for your private life (Fig. 5.5).

In addition, self-selected structures can be helpful, e.g. clear "time pockets" which you define for yourself once and then periodically keep free. Or the everyday orientation of "after ...pm I stop work for the day and no longer open emails", and so on.

Of course, you can also use a different system for classification – simply find something that suits you. One of the most famous is the Eisenhower Matrix, which dates back to the World War General and later US President (Eisenhower 1954). All tasks are divided into urgent/not urgent and important and unimportant. The "important combined with urgent" must be done immediately, the "unimportant combined with not urgent" can be omitted.

The Eisenhower Matrix was created for work under time pressure in military and political everyday hustle and bustle. In my opinion, it is only partially suitable for ADHD, since the required degree the tasks should be completed is not taken into account. And the latter in particular often represents one of the main difficulties for ADHDers.

5.2.5.5 A Budget for Work Projects with Passion

ADHDers make associations in an unchecked way and produce many ideas. Most of them are not feasible, either for reasons of time and energy, or because one is employed to do something else, or because an idea is not practical. Concentrating on your core work becomes boring however, especially when exciting ideas continually appear. Abandoning your own ideas can be frustrating and exhausting.

Here, too, a budget—which you do not need to reconsider every time—can be helpful. A budget with which I define the annual effort for special projects which *I allow myself* to expend, in order to implement them. This results in two advantages:

- Firstly, the budget makes it easier to select your own special projects in a targeted way.
- Secondly, reducing things to a small number of defined projects increases the chance of sticking to them and even bringing them to fruition. And to do this satisfactorily, not necessarily perfectly.

In this way, you are not running after every idea without having realised even one of them at the end. Rather, you give yourself the opportunity periodically to implement your own interesting ideas. Over the years, you can build up a considerable number of implemented projects in this way, as a marker of your own achievements, including the resulting satisfaction.

> **Encore**
> Beware of wanting to select the single best idea! You will never finish selecting the absolutely perfect one. Reach for any of the reasonably good ideas that can be implemented under your given private and professional circumstances. And one that is also quite realistic in terms of its scope. If necessary, you can also decide by drawing lots.

You can also use the graphic below for visualisation, in which the non-ADHD and ADHD variants are shown overdrawn on the basis of the path from A to B. As a third possibility, a deliberately balanced (but not boringly mediocre) controlled optimal idea is outlined (Fig. 5.6).

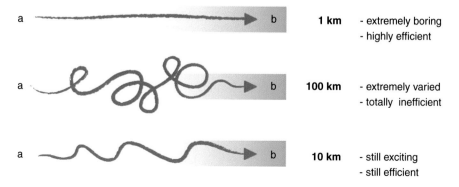

Fig. 5.6 Two extremes compared to the best possible

5.2.5.6 "Guilt-Free Time Pockets"

I don't know any ADHDer who doesn't have times when nothing gets done. Absolutely nothing. Despite having a long to-do list of tasks and a lack of time. At one point you're sitting on the couch, eating crisps or chocolate, watching endless series, wanting to finally relax, having an increasingly guilty conscience, therefore stuffing yourself all the more, drinking alcohol on top of this and getting increasingly bogged down.

Until you're totally exhausted.

Despite all the planning, getting an overview of the situation and the tasks, you sometimes completely forget that it is just as important to recover. Above all, to let the brain recover.

Of course, orgies of eating, drinking and series-watching lasting several days make no sense. If only for the reason that, if they proceed as described above, they do not offer recuperation but ultimately contribute to your exhaustion. Because having a guilty conscience is an absolute energy guzzler for the human brain.

It is therefore important that you always plan time pockets where you can relax. A proportion of these time pockets should also be reserved for letting go completely. And also for doing what I described at the beginning, i.e. a temporary existence as a couch potato. However, with two main differences. Namely:

- The act of letting go and becoming a couch potato should be based on your own clear decision, and does not arise accidentally or because of procrastination. If it is your own decision, you give yourself the task, so to speak, of letting go, which prevents you from getting a guilty conscience.
- You decide to let go for a pre-defined time frame, i.e. in no case for an endless period of time. This previously defined restriction is necessary in order not to "lose yourself", and ultimately end up reproaching yourself.

In this way, the effect of a letting go can produce a 180° change. The main factor here is that you can enjoy "chilling" without a guilty conscience. It is a useful—indeed necessary—time-out for the brain. In this way, it does actually lead to recuperation.

5.2.5.7 Cultivating Relationships Consciously (Without Bootlicking)

One of the big energy guzzlers at work is strained working relationships. Of course, the advice that you should simply cultivate good relationships is no use to anyone. It's easier said than done.

However, when dealing with emerging tensions, it can be helpful to ask yourself *quietly* a few questions about how the situation came about.

The point of this is definitely not to blame yourself for everything, protect the other person, nor "worm your way in" by bootlicking. No, it's just about staying aware:

- I could be right with my "spontaneous" assessment that the other person rejects me, has dropped me in it, is nasty, etc.

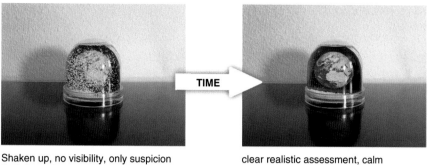

Shaken up, no visibility, only suspicion   clear realistic assessment, calm
Activity reduces visibility even more   **Action is now very possible**

Fig. 5.7 Enhanced "snow globe effect" with ADHD: fewer filters → more data

- But I could also have perceived something in a negatively focussed or distorted way.
- Or I could have accidentally triggered a negative reaction in the other person, by an impulsive statement/action that was incomprehensible to them, or by an intrusion into their area of responsibility.
- etc.

As you know, it is especially difficult to ask yourself these questions in such situations quietly and to take your time. But this is exactly what is necessary. The image of a snow globe helps to explain this. Shaking it (arguing; immediately deciding your opinion; etc.) does not bring a clearer view inside the globe—on the contrary! The flakes are only stirred up even more. It is only by waiting that the clear view returns (Fig. 5.7).

Sometimes it also makes sense to get an outside opinion from someone you trust. Not with the idea that the outsider is always right. Rather, because comparing your own assessment with the opinion of an outsider allows you to get a true-to-reality relativisation. Very often, workplace conflicts with ADHD are caused by misunderstandings and the increased emotional reactions created by negative hyperfocus.

In this context, it can be a relief for you to tell your colleagues that you occasionally get carried away. Whether it's with excitement or feeling offended. And that then you would be quite happy for them to slow you down—of course, only with velvet gloves.

5.2.6 Burnout-Protective Factors of ADHD?

At the end of this subchapter on chronic stress and burnout, I would like to mention that ADHD also has some sides that can protect you a little from burnout.

5.2.6.1 Capacity for Enthusiasm

For a start, there is the capacity for enthusiasm, a positive hyperfocus which can also last for long periods of time if the person has high intrinsic interest. This mobilises existing energies, especially when the work is flowing and thereby motivating you.

> **Encore**
> On the other hand, there is the danger—and every ADHDer knows this—of overexerting yourself and getting wound up in the task. This usually only becomes problematic when you get stuck in your work (or at most, your private life collapses). Two reactions are typical:
>
> • Reflexively, in an attempt to overcome the blockade, you end up expending even more energy. It is important to recognise this reflex and consciously slow it down. Otherwise, the burnout-protective effect of the capacity for enthusiasm gradually turns into one that is burnout-promoting.
> • Getting stuck triggers a negative hyperfocus that leads to resignation and wanting to give up. Obviously, this reaction also increases the risk of exhaustion and burnout. In this case, follow the procedure under Sect. 6.4.

The capacity for enthusiasm through positive hyperfocus contributes significantly to the ability to bounce back.

5.2.6.2 Jobs That You Can Highly Identify with, and Those with a Strong Structure

Another occupational factor that can protect ADHDers from burnout is an early-developed coping mechanism, in which external factors are particularly strongly used for orientation.

These types of ADHDers can orientate themselves very well in structures and companies that offer them jobs *that they can highly identify with* (Felfe 2008). This high identification level has an energy-saving effect, as permanent thinking about the meaning of the work or about the working structure becomes obsolete.

The same is true in structures that have *great power externally*—always provided that the authority behind it is accepted by the ADHDer concerned. These include, for example, the police, the military and monasteries, but also successful market leaders whose position is so powerful that they have a similarly absolute abundance of power for employees. It should be emphasised however: this power is neither positive nor negative per se.

Focussing strongly on external structures hereby has a high energy-saving and thus burnout-protective effect. The externally provided guidelines are followed on "autopilot" so to speak, making it possible to achieve high performance over a long period of time.

Encore

At the same time, a danger also lurks in this protective factor. If someone has developed a coping strategy with an orientation towards external structures, there is an increased risk that the person concerned—quasi as a side effect of their coping mechanism—will resort to increasing dependencies. These can be submissive relationships, as occurred in certain companies during the hype preceding the subprime crisis of 2008, but also radical political groups of any persuasion, in criminal gangs, fundamentalist-religious groups as well as dependencies on doctors and therapists who have a guru-like effect.

The risk is especially high if there is no awareness of this danger—as is the case with all dangers.

5.2.6.3 Shorter Perception Duration

Under Sect. 4.3 I wrote about psychodynamic difficulties (earlier known as neuroses). In other words, difficulties that are based on unprocessed experiences and feelings in the past. Such difficulties are very common in people in general and can cause an enormous amount of suffering. Among other things, they consume a lot of mental energy. They increase the risk of burnout.

Statistically speaking (this does not apply to everyone!) ADHDers experience significantly more stressful situations when they are growing up (Barkley 2004), which could contribute to psychodynamic developments. But it seems to be the case that despite this, there is no corresponding, proportionally increased rate of psychodynamic difficulties. This could mean that ADHD can have a certain neurosis-protective effect and, consequently can protect you to a certain extent from this specific burnout factor.

Encore

Hypothetically, one can assume that in ADHD, many situations and the feelings they trigger are stored less prominently, and are pushed out of the perceptual focus more quickly by other experiences. As a result, these areas would trigger less unconscious fear, which would explain a lower development of the psychodynamic (neurotic), self-destructive defence mechanisms.

On the other hand, if negative hyperfocus occurs during a stressful experience, a particularly strong traumatisation (formerly referred to as "neurotisation") may also develop.

5.3   Acute Stress: Emergency Benefit with ADHD

Acute stress is not necessarily bad. It can make life attractive and exciting in the best sense. In addition, acute stressful situations, accidents and all kinds of emergencies are part of our life anyway.

This sub-chapter is about a tangible benefit of ADHD (yes, when I wrote about the advantages, it wasn't just empty words!). This special advantage can sometimes also have side effects, but these can be prevented. But don't forget: this is only if you understand for yourself how ADHD works.

5.3.1   Advantage

It has long been known that ADHDers are usually more helpful than average (Ryffel-Rawak 2007), and that their performance in accidents, disasters and emergency situations is usually exceptional.

Among excellent emergency helpers and emergency doctors, you will find a striking number of ADHDers. ADHDers are also strongly represented in other hectic professions that require improvisational talent and have phases that are acutely stressful (police, journalism, stock exchange trading, show business, etc.).

Why is this so?

5.3.1.1 Short Version

The adrenaline surge in an emergency situation provides the ADHDer with a short-term activation of the filter. As a result, his filter function increases much more in comparison to a non-ADHDer with the same adrenaline surge. The ADHDer rises above the "fog line" so to speak, gets a clear overview and feels secure. In addition, compared to the non-ADHDer, he can benefit from his better training condition in dealing with unclear situations, owing to his own life experiences.

5.3.1.2 Detailed Version

Let's go back to the basics. In ADHD, there is less dopamine and noradrenaline available at certain places in the brain (Arnsten et al. 1996), where they activate a kind of automatic pre-filter (see Chap. 3). Without this pre-filter, there is always a surplus of information and one's own thoughts, which causes a kind of "data fog". For areas with which you are not particularly familiar, you therefore have trouble gaining the "big picture"—an overview of things.

Let's illustrate this in a schematic diagram (Fig. 5.8), in which the horizontal branch represents the available noradrenaline or adrenaline, respectively, and the vertical branch represents the corresponding activation of the automatic pre-filter for information (in other words, the degree of clarity).

Non-ADHDers have a higher activation of the filter in everyday life due to the higher noradrenaline availability. Their starting point on the curve in Fig. 5.8 is therefore relatively far to the right, as well as already quite high. In the case of an emergency-related adrenaline surge, a certain increase in clear-sightedness is the result, but the corresponding additional benefit (threshold benefit) is minimal.

This contrasts with the ADHDer:

- His everyday quantity of available noradrenaline is relatively low; on the curve he lies far to the left—and at the bottom. If he gets the same adrenaline surge as

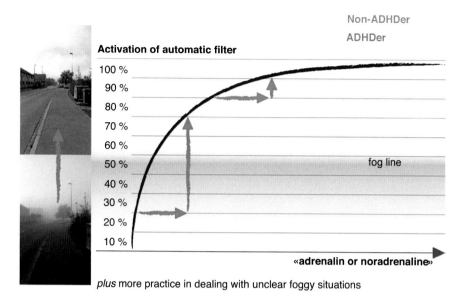

Fig. 5.8 ADHD advantage in an emergency or acute stress situation

a non-ADHDer, he therefore benefits greatly from the increase in filtering. In one fell swoop, the view clears, similarly to when fog disappears. In one fell swoop, you can see everything more clearly distinguishable than you usually see it. Despite the stress of the emergency situation, this is also experienced in a positive and liberating way. Because as soon as I see something clearly, I can get started, and finally feel all the real potential that I have.

- In addition, the fact that ADHDers are forced to deal with unclear situations much more often during their lives, due to the "data fog", plays a major role in helping them deal with emergency situations. They learn how to deal with uncertainty, mostly without being aware of this. As a result, most of them have exceptional experience and above-average practice in dealing with unclear situations. This is enormously valuable in emergency situations, because the essence of every emergency situation is that it is unclear at first.
- Yes, and the fundamentally greater breadth of association in ADHDers as well, which—because it has been consolidated by use—can also be helpful, despite the adrenaline-activated pre-filter.

Multidimensional research, focussing on understanding the meaning of the functional processes involved, would provide rich scientific opportunities for any scientist interested in taking on this task!

Encore

One can illustrate the ADHD processes in acute stressful situations very well by using a comparison from everyday life: the rev counter in your car.

In the case of non-ADHDers, the dial is fixed in green/orange/red. As the engine speed increases, you are constantly approaching the load limits.

In the case of ADHDers, the dial is not fixed. At the low speeds of less exciting everyday life, the green range is narrow, you are almost moving up to the orange area, if not even into the red. But if the engine revs up, because things are getting exciting and the adrenaline is flowing, the dial also turns up. The red range shifts from 4000 rpm to over 20,000 rpm, while the green range becomes very wide. In other words, you can only really get into the green range at high speed.

This roughly corresponds to the behaviour of Formula 1 cars. At a rotational speed that is normal for everyday cars, the engine cuts out. It only runs smoothly when the revs are pushed up into a range that the engines of everyday cars would not survive.

ADHD therefore means quite an advantage in stressful situations. This is useful to know. Because, owing to their perception of self-worth which is impaired for many reasons, many ADHDers do not trust themselves with exciting professional paths that they could actually master perfectly. Yes, for which they might even be predestined.

Knowing about these advantages of ADHD is of great importance for companies and for society as a whole. The potential is ready and waiting, if you know how to use it.

5.3.2   Possible Side Effects of the Emergency Benefit

I have met quite a number of ADHDers who, despite their "emergency benefit", ultimately "disintegrated" because of it. This can happen especially when the person concerned notices the positive effect of adrenaline kicks, but does not know why he reacts with so much clarity. And even more important, if he does not know why he does not have this clarity all the time in other areas of life.

Here is a selection of typical, possible side effects, which can be prevented with the appropriate knowledge of the background situation:

5.3.2.1 Emotional Rollercoaster Leads to Self-Doubt and Professional Resignation

Severe self-doubt, chronic fear of overload, exhaustion and professional resignation are often described by ADHDers who otherwise cope superbly in an emergency profession.

Why is this so? Let's take a look at the processes *after* a super performance in an emergency situation.

As long as the adrenaline surge lasts, the person experiences a clear view of the situation, has no trouble with the assessment and can make the most of all their knowledge and skills. Of course, this is an uplifting feeling compared to the everyday life of an ADHDer. It triggers well-deserved satisfaction and self-confidence.

If the adrenaline level drops after the emergency situation, the perception becomes blurred again, the awareness of one's own abilities is reduced. In brief: the "fog" returns.

In this fog, the person's overview of the completed actions in particular also recedes. The emergency doctor suddenly asks himself, "Did I actually stop the bleeding, or did I just want to do it, but missed it in the hustle and bustle?" And to make matters worse, he may lose his clear time association of the overall event.

This *experienced* course of events can understandably lead to doubts about one's own value and competence. It triggers fear; in the example above on whether the patient has been treated correctly, or whether he is bleeding to death internally. The need for security and a sense of responsibility lead to control actions. The doctor described above goes to check the patient far too often, ultimately to reassure himself and not the patient. This consumes a lot of time and energy and leads to inefficiency.

If the person in the above situation still knows that he or she has mastered the emergency well, the renewed loss of orientation in the fog manifests itself in such a way that the doctor fears that he or she has only done the right thing by chance and that the next emergency will certainly not be manageable. This develops into a fear of being overloaded, which leads to exhaustion, passivity and ultimately to professional resignation. The gifted emergency doctor ends up despondent as a bleary-eyed diagnostic coder in a hospital's bureaucratic back office.

5.3.2.2 Adrenaline Junkie at Work

In order to maintain the uplifting feeling from the adrenaline surge, the ADHDer seeks out challenging and even more risky tasks. The willingness to engage in professional risk behaviour increases, for example to perform risky operations, highly speculative financial transactions, or to "go it alone" as a police inspector, something which is popular in crime novels, etc. The boundary to criminal behaviour is not always respected here.

In other words: In the search for the professional adrenaline rush, the healthy balance is easily lost; you overexert yourself, crash, or burn out.

5.3.2.3 Adrenaline Junkie in Private Life

Others tend simply to continue the repeated adrenaline kicks into their private lives in order to experience more clarity and, above all, more of their potential there as well. This can be with risky sports, hectic party and sex life, legal and illegal drugs, extreme political activism or comparable activities (keywords "no risk no fun" or "yolo = you only live once"). This can easily result in an accident or another disaster.

Sometimes the fatigue resulting from such a risky and energy-consuming private life is enough to lead to a professional decline. If accidents, other complications or legal consequences occur, tragic outcomes can result.

Encore
Naturally I do not want to waggle a moralising index finger here. Anyone is free to pursue these activities—as long as they are legal—as they choose. Rather, I would like to point out that to achieve the effect that ADHDers are aiming for, this kind of risky, extreme and often addictive behaviour is unnecessary. To put it another way: you can have the same effect (without the risk of addiction and without practising "suicidal" behaviour) with less risk.

5.3.2.4 Private Passivity and Resignation
Of course, the opposite can also occur as a side effect of the emergency benefit and unfortunately every often:

A working day as an emotional rollercoaster: experiencing one's own top performance and then sinking into self-doubt is indeed enormously tiring. In everyday life (= for ADHDers, every single day or at least "just today" on a daily basis), all you want is retreat, peace, familiar TV series, beer, pizza and sweets. At least that's how it seems at the moment.

And yet, the dream of an active private life with activities, hobbies, an intense romantic relationship and a rich cultural and social life as well as recreational sports exists, it is true, but all efforts in this direction fail every day under the prerequisites described above.

5.3.3   Suggested Solutions for the Side Effects of the Emergency Benefit

ADHDers can usually avoid the side effects of the emergency benefit by being aware of the functional processes of ADHD and applying their characteristics to their own situation.

The key here is to be able to assess one's own strengths and weaknesses. It's worth consciously comparing yourself with others, in other words, doing something that psychiatrists and psychologists otherwise often advise against doing (see also section "Compare Yourself Consciously with Others"). But *this* comparison is not about competing or degrading the other person, nor about power intrigues. The aim is to get a realistic assessment of yourself. Here, "realistic" often proves to be "better than expected" for ADHDers. In this way, you become more confident in your abilities and also more assertive in a constructive sense.

As a rule, one usually becomes *less* arrogant!

Encore

Without these "assured" comparisons, ADHDers run a great risk of always seeing themselves in a worse light than they actually are (see also Sect. 7.1). Nevertheless, the reverse is also true: in some situations, an ADHDer also realises that he can be superior to others. It's just that, if you don't have enough lasting confidence in yourself, you will end up holding back excessively. Sooner or later you get frustrated, because you don't earn the merits for your abilities in the way that other people do. You get jealous. From envy, combined with self-doubt and selective experience of one's own excellence, it is only a very small step to a generally arrogant attitude.

This is why it is often the case that ADHD is confused with narcissistic pathologies.

The rule of thumb for distinguishing the ADHD behaviour I have just described from pathological narcissistic behaviour:

- If you admit your own mistake to a narcissist, then he will come to the conclusion of his own alleged superiority and immediately abuse it in order to position himself condescendingly and powerfully against you. In pathological narcissism, it is always about power.
- When admitting a mistake, ADHDers, on the other hand, tend to react by saying something like "not so bad, could have happened to me". Often, ADHDers are even embarrassed when the other person apologises for a mistake. Fundamentally, ADHD is not about power.

5.4 Innovation Advantage of People with ADHD: With Possible Side Effects

To dispel some illusions: not all ADHDers are particularly innovative.

Having a good practical or theoretical intelligence is always a necessary prerequisite for inventiveness. The distribution of intelligence in ADHD is the same as in the rest of the population (Kaplan et al. 2000). For ADHDers who have good intelligence (this can also include those whose school career was less than outstanding!), the ADHD mode of operation offers a few additional advantages (White 2019).

Here, I would like to highlight three factors in particular. They are naturally based on the same neurobiological factors. It has proven useful to keep a special eye on these three principles in practical, everyday life with ADHD.

5.4.1 Factor 1: Positive Effect of the ADHD Learning Mode (Learning Curve)

Under Sect. 5.1, I describe how the ADHD condition influences the way ADHDers absorb information. Once again, I would like to emphasise that this description concerns the native state, in other words, without the coping mechanisms developed during our lives. The type of unfiltered absorption and the resulting learning curve can not only initially cause a slowdown, but also produce a positive follow-up effect.

As an advantage, it leads to the fact that an ADHDer who studies a particular field for a long time, and ideally is also interested in it, acquires significantly more knowledge in this field than an equally intelligent non-ADHD person with about the same length of experience. The ADHDer collects considerably more detailed knowledge.

From the moment of the sharp increase in the learning curve, this detailed information is no longer stored individually, but has been recorded in its inherent functional context.

When it comes to reforms, further and new developments as well as unexpected problems in this field, the ADHDer has decisive advantage:

- Owing to the reduced, automatic pre-filtering, a much greater amount of detailed knowledge is available.
- The existing data are stored less rigidly in the usual, theoretically formalised categories, but more in the functional contexts inherent in the field itself. In other words, they are less dependent on externally determined views and therefore more flexible.

The meaning is clear. The probability of finding unusual solutions quickly is higher.

Of course, sometimes incorrect connections can be made. A partnership in which an ADHDer has the freedom to innovate but an equally strong non-ADHDer is placed at his side on an equal footing would therefore be an ideal situation. However, this kind of arrangement would only be constructive with the prerequisite that the two respect each other.

Case Study 9
The Inspired Developer Who Had to Repeat a Year in Primary School
When I met Paul, he was already almost 60 years old. A short time earlier, after a stay in hospital, he had been given the diagnosis of ADHD.

Paul showed an impressive life journey. In primary school his performance was so poor, he had to repeat a year. After that, he only just managed the lowest qualification at the end of his compulsory schooling. With the help of a friend, he just about passed an apprenticeship as a mason. For lack of alternatives, he joined the military, where he stayed for two years, making it to rank of sergeant.

After that, he surprised everyone who knew him. He completed his general high school graduation in record time via the adult education route and successfully studied mechanical engineering at ETH Zurich (one of the top ten universities in the world, would you believe!). He then worked for various companies in all sorts of countries around the world. Despite outstanding achievements, his career was repeatedly slowed down by self-doubt, depressive phases and not infrequently also by conflicts with superiors and colleagues. At least, thanks to the support of his wife, he was always able to pick himself up again.

But with one special work location, everything was different. After the end of the Cold War, he worked for a few years for a company that had to set up several production facilities for a corporation in a vast area east of the Ural Mountains in Russia. His job was characterised by complex questions of a technical nature, also in relation to the local conditions, both climatic and social. He often had to commute between locations which were several hundred kilometres apart. They were eternal car trips, which he usually took with his direct supervisor.

On these trips, he developed numerous ideas, found dozens of unusual solutions, came up with a lot of innovations, which he simply described openly in conversation with his boss.

- It was important for Paul to be occupied at the wheel, so as not to get nervous and unfocussed from being passive as a passenger on the endless journey.
- It was equally important that his boss recognised the quality of the exploratory associations he was making and his conceptualising thinking, while himself holding back during the conversation, and merely keeping the development process on the right tracks by asking specific questions.
- It was also crucial that the boss wrote down these ideas. Something that Paul could not have managed to do after such trips.
- And of course, the integrity of the boss, who recorded the noted ideas as achievements of Paul, was also central to the further, motivated cooperation.

This was the happiest time in Paul's professional life. The conditions were ideal for his ingenious inventiveness. Unfortunately, it did not last. After the end of the assignment, he returned to Switzerland and to a working environment which was far less favourable for him. Again there were conflicts, and gloomy phases, which later led to a deadlocked chronic-depressive state of exhaustion, with a far-reaching limitation on his ability to work.

Unfortunately, hospital stays, various outpatient treatments, job coaching and support measures for occupational reintegration could not change anything.

This was a pity because if he and the companies he had worked for had had the appropriate knowledge, his career path would have been much more successful. He and his family would have suffered less. His employers would have benefitted more from him.

But at least Paul got a sense of satisfaction in understanding why he was brilliantly inventive and could use his potential in some situations and not in others. He understood that it was by no means due to lack of motivation or laziness. So, his "years east of the Ural Mountains" remained at least a happy memory, since he had been able to find peace with the subsequent difficult years, at least in retrospect.

5.4.2   Factor 2: Highly Trained Ability to Extrapolate

Let's imagine a small child with ADHD who has an excellent level of intelligence. With uninteresting things, he is quickly distracted, and does not pay attention to everything. He has several options for dealing with this characteristic of his personality, which is impractical in everyday life.

Case Study 10

The Personnel Manager Who, as a Girl, Learned Fast—And Almost Too Well

Alice is a young, successful HR manager. When she started school, she was very interested, both in the school material and in the new colleagues. She found detailed information about homework, organisational instructions and the like less exciting. She was quickly distracted, only half-listened and didn't pay attention to everything.

As her first coping mechanism with this awkward circumstance, Alice took advantage of her own powers of observation. If she heard an instruction twice in succession, she would be distracted at different places each time and would miss various parts of both instructions. She realised that she did not have all the information she needed. So, she would listen with big eyes to the corresponding instructions of the teacher. As soon as he had finished, she would ask innocently, "could you tell me that again?"

Technically, this coping mechanism was effective, but socially it had the opposite effect. The teacher, understandably, perceived this as ranging from rude to provocative. There were also tit-for-tat responses on the part of the teacher.

In short, this coping mechanism is effective, but its side effects are significantly higher than the benefits.

Alice reacted quickly to this negative experience. She stopped asking. She tried to derive the totality of the instructions from the fragments of information instead.

Her second coping mechanism therefore consisted of extrapolating. As her thinking ability was very good, she quickly achieved a high degree of accuracy. This ability is also extremely useful to Alice as an adult woman in many ways.

Why on earth should this learning be "almost too good"?

The key word is "almost" here. Of course, this extrapolating thinking is fantastic. Nevertheless, it has side effects, which I explain in the text below.

Most smart ADHDers use their powers of reasoning when they miss information given to them due to the fact that they were distracted. They learn to extrapolate at an early age. They are highly trained in this ability and have a clear advantage over equally intelligent non-ADHDers. However, it's important to pay attention to some possible circumstances and disadvantages:

- Since the development of derivation or extrapolation takes place involuntarily, most ADHDers are not aware that they are significantly more practised in this than comparable non-ADHDers.
- They therefore assume that this ability is normal and average. Anyone can do it! This is a logical but incorrect assumption that can lead to various misunderstandings.
- If you start a long explanation to an ADHDer who is highly practised in this way, then he usually understands very quickly what you are leading to. But if the ADHDer in question is unaware of his extrapolating ability, he gets the impression that the other person thinks he is stupid. Why else would this person want to tell me the completely obvious facts at great length?
- As a result, the corresponding ADHDer tends to interrupt his opposite number twice as quickly. Possibly, even with the offended-reproachful attitude of, "you probably think I'm stupid".
- If they are not aware of the background of these abilities, ADHDers can easily come to the misjudgement over time that "the others" are generally not very intelligent. That can be devastating, as we will see later in this chapter.

Nevertheless, the highly trained skill in extrapolating is one of the most amazing and—especially professionally—most valuable qualities of bright ADHDers.

5.4.3   Factor 3: Positive Hyperfocus (Positive Tunnel Vision)

In the context of the explanations about the functional system of ADHD above (Sect. 3.2.1), I mentioned positive hyperfocus. When an ADHDer has a genuine interest in something, he concentrates on it better and longer than a comparable non-ADHDer.

> **Encore**
> What I mean by genuine interest is best explained by this example: I am interested in being able to speak Chinese, but I have no interest in learning Chinese. Therefore, I will never be able to speak Chinese. My daughter, on the other hand, has had a genuine interest in learning Russian since childhood. So, she started doing it early. In the meantime, her Russian is quite advanced and allows her to travel easily in Russia and Ukraine.

Now it so happens that cognitive ability is by no means limited *within* hyperfocus; rather, all thoughts, associations and possible combination variants are very quickly compared with each other and thought out. Humanity owes numerous extraordinary achievements and inventions to this ADHD-related positive hyperfocus—combined with the great breadth of association also given within the hyperfocus.

This is another tangible advantage that you have as an ADHDer. It can be used professionally very well, ultimately in every profession. But here, too, it is important to understand your own way of operating, and to recognise how you should apply this *"nuclear power of ADHD"*. Without harming yourself—or causing harm to others.

In order to illustrate this, I'll relate the story of a mechanical and production engineer with ADHD, who worked in the field of bakery production.

Case Study 11
Brilliant but a Loser: The Expat in a Swiss Biscuit Factory
François was a gifted Belgian engineer with ADHD in his mid-30s. He was employed by a large company known for its social policies, but where the management had no knowledge regarding ADHD.

In the production of the traditional *Guetsli* biscuits, the task was to analyse the outdated production method, evaluate possibilities for new ways and ideally propose a tangible process and procedure. There was already a favoured proposal from the previous crew.

After a short time, François realised that this proposal had serious disadvantages. He thought about everything anew from scratch and from other than the usual perspectives. He developed a new production process that was simpler, cheaper and safer. Yes, it even offered the prospect of improved quality of the biscuits made using it.

François enthusiastically talked about his idea with the other engineers, other employees involved and his superiors in the management. He dispelled anyone's objections at lightening speed. He explained everything in detail and presented comparative offers already obtained from tool suppliers. He almost made people dizzy with his talking.

And he sensed a general feeling of hesitation extending to outright rejection. He became increasingly irritated and reacted in a manner ranging from casual to condescending. After some time, he began to display a cynical, arrogant behaviour. His position became increasingly isolated. Shortly after his ideas were definitely rejected, he was dismissed and received an unsatisfactory job reference.

Six months later, the company implemented the proposals he had developed, which were rejected at the time. François himself did not reap the benefit of his idea.

However, the company could not benefit further from his inventiveness either. Ultimately, unfortunately, it was a lose-lose situation for everyone.

Unfortunately, such stories abound among ADHDers. Let's take a step-by-step look at how this situation came about. This will help us to see how such disasters can be prevented in the future.

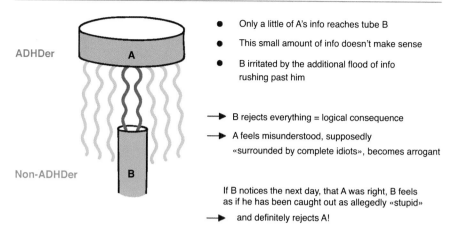

ADHDer

- Only a little of A's info reaches tube B
- This small amount of info doesn't make sense
- B irritated by the additional flood of info rushing past him

→ B rejects everything = logical consequence

→ A feels misunderstood, supposedly «surrounded by complete idiots», becomes arrogant

Non-ADHDer

If B notices the next day, that A was right, B feels as if he has been caught out as allegedly «stupid»

→ and definitely rejects A!

Fig. 5.9 Diagram: side effect of positive hyperfocus when your counterpart is "swamped" by your ADHD ideas

5.4.4   Which Prerequisites Intensify the Risk Potential?

When an intelligent ADHDer...

- knows a particular field well
- is interested in it
- has unchecked thought associations
- has developed an idea, is enthusiastic → **gets into positive hyperfocus**
- and as an "encore", has reduced impulse control

...then the risk of communication difficulties with his environment is very high.

This applies even more so if the environment is long-established and there are old established rights, as was the case with the traditional company he used to work for.

When these conditions coincide, the result is typically an escalating order of events (see Fig. 5.9). Neither side is fundamentally behaving in an "evil" way. In both cases, their reactions are plausible and understandable. However, typical yet different misunderstandings arise in both cases.

5.4.5   Suggested Solutions for the Side Effects of the Innovation Advantage

If you are familiar with how your ADHD works, then you can fundamentally remain attached to your own sense of value. In addition, you can better understand that someone who cannot immediately follow your enthusiastic ideas—presented at a fast pace—is not necessarily stupid. It is even possible that they are more intelligent than you. In any case, it's important that you don't swamp them *too fast with too much at once.*

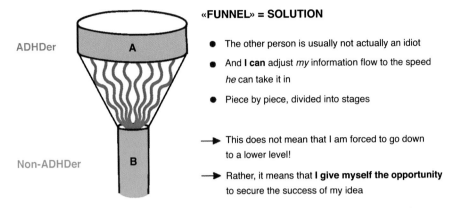

ADHDer

Non-ADHDer

«FUNNEL» = SOLUTION

● The other person is usually not actually an idiot

● And **I can** adjust *my* information flow to the speed *he* can take it in

● Piece by piece, divided into stages

→ This does not mean that I am forced to go down to a lower level!

→ Rather, it means that **I give myself the opportunity** to secure the success of my idea

Fig. 5.10 Solution for the side effect of positive hyperfocus

If you really understand this (not only intellectually, but also emotionally), then you are not just "adapting to an idiot" if you slowly and step by step, at first only outline the rough outlines of your ideas. Rather, you give the other person the chance to take in and engage with your idea in the first place.

At a later stage, they will be more receptive to the more complex correlations and details. They may even see suggestions for improvement that they dare to put forward (Fig. 5.10).

Technically, you can use all known methods to "rein yourself in". But only one of these procedures will really suit you. Not everyone can focus on their own points of reference, consciously grasped in advance, by means of a symbolic object (e.g. a stone in your trouser pocket, which you can take in your hand and thus physically feel). It's a matter of trying things out and paying attention to your own ideas. It is worth discussing this with your partner, in self-help groups or with a doctor, therapist or coach.

I especially recommend the method of speaking deliberately slowly, although not sluggishly, which can be learned. This means that you cannot say as much you would say otherwise, if your thoughts were unchecked. And it automatically means that you need be selective in choosing the thoughts you will express. At the same time, slowing down also gives you more time to filter the things that are relevant.

This makes it easier to give a presentation which people can understand and get an overview of. It takes a little practice—and perhaps you will need to overcome some resistance to the idea. But it offers a very good "return on investment".

In brief: For a discussion in which the other person should have the chance to follow what I am saying, an andante is much better than a prestissimo. Occasionally, when someone is unstoppable in their flow of speech, I bring out a very loud and annoyingly ticking metronome and, with a twinkle in my eye, set it ticking at the high speaking rhythm of my opposite number. The conversation instantly settles down again, meaning that I can switch off the terrible ticking again.

References

Arnsten AF, Steere JC, Hunt RD. The contribution of alpha 2-noradrenergic mechanism of prefrontal cortical cognitive function. Potential significance for attention-deficit hyperactivity disorder. Arch Gen Psychiatry. 1996;53:448–55.

Barkley RA. Adolescents with attention-deficit/hyperactivity disorder: an overview of empirically based treatments. J Psychiatr Pract. 2004;10(1):39–56.

Burisch M. Das Burnout-Syndrom. Berlin: Springer; 1989.

Eisenhower DD. Address at the second assembly of the World Council of Churches. Illinois: Evaston; 1954.

Felfe J. Mitarbeiterbindung. Göttingen: Hogrefe; 2008.

Kaplan BJ, Crawford SG, Dewey DM, Fisher GC. The IQs of children with ADHD are normally distributed. J Learn Disabil. 2000;33:425–32.

Lennie P. The cost of cortical computation. Curr Biol. 2003;13:493–7.

Neuhaus C. Lass mich, doch verlass mich nicht. Munich: Deutscher Taschenbuchverlag; 2005.

Ryffel-Rawak D. ADHS bei Erwachsenen. Bern: Huber; 2007.

Selye H. A syndrome produced by diverse nocuous agents. Nature. 1936;138:32.

White H. The creativity of ADHD. Sci Am (Springer Nature America). 2019.

The Curse of Negative Hyperfocus (Negative Tunnel Vision)

6

This chapter deals with negative hyperfocus and its reinforcing influences. In my experience, these quantitative effects are more significant in ADHD than the qualitative distortions that can also occur in negative hyperfocus (see also the explanations about quantitative and qualitative hyperfocus under Sect. 3.2.1).

Negative hyperfocus is responsible for an enormous amount of suffering and failure in the working lives of ADHDers. It therefore needs special attention, especially in an occupational context.

6.1 The Absolutely Worst ADHD Cowpats

Unfortunately, the phenomenon of hyperfocus doesn't just exist with great things and genuine interest. It can also occur when something goes wrong (Lachenmeier 2014). If a negative stimulus (criticism from other people, a disappointment, one's own mistake, or even a mistake made by another person, etc.) attracts attention, then the field of perception narrows excessively—this is the definition of negative hyperfocus. One-sided excessive emotional reactions are the result (Neuhaus 2005).

> **Encore**
> Naturally non-ADHDers can also slip into negative hyperfocus. However, this usually requires much stronger stimuli than is the case for ADHDers.

It is devastating that the constricted view of negative hyperfocus is perceived subjectively and emotionally as being allegedly the whole picture. Consequently, you can be completely convinced that at that moment you are seeing the (allegedly) entire truth.

© The Author(s), under exclusive license to Springer Nature
Switzerland AG 2023
H. Lachenmeier, *ADHD and Success at Work*,
https://doi.org/10.1007/978-3-031-13437-1_6

If the perception is limited to the relevant section of your tunnel vision, then you can no longer relativise the situation by comparing it to the overall circumstances of what has just happened or what was said. Similarly, as long as people are in negative hyperfocus, they no longer have any perception of their overall value to compensate them; in other words: all their abilities, qualities and achievements.

The consequence of this is:

- The situation will be **perceived as more extreme and assessed more radically**. For example, instead of a lack of sympathy, you suspect that you have been totally rejected; or instead of neutral criticism of details, you think you are experiencing a complete devaluation of your overall performance; or instead of thinking "I made an unimportant mistake", you think you are a total failure; etc.
- The **emotional reaction is correspondingly greatly intensified**. For example, instead of feeling mild annoyance, you fly into a rage; instead of being a little critical of yourself, you feel like an absolutely worthless loser; etc.
- The **impulses associated with your heightened feelings are greatly amplified accordingly** as a result, controlling them becomes more difficult.
- Your subsequent **options for action turn out to be excessive and exaggerated**; you attack your opposite number directly, verbally or physically; or you quit your job immediately under protest or possibly while making accusations about yourself.
- The result is an ugly **escalation situation**.

As long as you are trapped in negative hyperfocus, there seem to be only two possibilities:

- **Either** you attack the other person immediately or you defend yourself to the hilt. The idea behind this is that your respect or your self-worth is guaranteed only if you can assert yourself immediately or refute the criticism.
- **Or** you accept the criticism as justified, but as you are in a state of completely negative hyperfocus, this would mean that you (allegedly) have absolutely "no value"—probably the worst possible condition. Instant depression and even a suicidal tendency can be the result.

Due to these circumstances, ADHDers are often regarded as been incapable of taking criticism (Claus et al. 2005). This is only true to a limited extent, namely only if a negative hyperfocus has been triggered.

Encore
In my experience, the following applies: if at the point when ADHDers are criticised, they are given respect that is *perceivable at exactly the same moment*, then ADHDers are usually *better* (!) able to accept justified criticism than non-ADHDers.

Taking this ADHD functionality into consideration is of central importance during collaboration in a work setting (and of course also in private life). In particular, it means that ADHDers do not have to be "handled with kid gloves".

However, the respect mentioned above must be genuine and honest. Paternalistic shoulder-patting or sugar-coated platitudes do not work and can be counterproductive.

6.2   First and Second Wave of Negative Hyperfocus

The order of events is often as follows: in the first wave you rear up wildly, then fight back, defend yourself excessively and attack the others.

After some time, the hyperfocus begins to dissolve to a certain extent

As the tunnel vision gradually clears, your field of vision expands, as a result of which a different state of suffering threatens to engulf you, because you realise that you have overreacted. Regret and shame are consistently felt. This realisation and the associated feelings are followed by the second wave of negative hyperfocus, namely your own overreaction. Regret and shame become overpoweringly great, alongside a feeling of alleged worthlessness and depressive self-reproaches at the same time.

Encore
Quite frequently, ADHDers fall into the habit of making excessive apologies, repetitive regrets, pleas for forgiveness and vows of improvement when the second wave of negative hyperfocus occurs. I recommend that you avoid doing this.

A serious apology, however, should be clear, short and straightforward.

The course of events with a second wave becomes more likely to happen, the stronger the previous escalation was.

In any case, negative hyperfocus isn't helpful for anyone—neither the ADHDer, nor their superiors or subordinates, nor their colleagues at the same level and certainly not the partners in other companies or clients.

Negative hyperfocus leads to wasted energy, wasted time, wasted goodwill, wasted social benefits and is probably the biggest sh… in ADHD.

Encore
These courses of events with negative hyperfocus must be taken into account in the topic of the "**mobbing**" of ADHDers at work. I have deliberately put the term mobbing between quotation marks because it is often no longer used in the original sense: when a group—a mob—bullies an individual for no reason.

Without wanting to attack ADHDers (and I am one of them myself) and defend "the others": honestly, it's annoying when someone in the team is offended too quickly, flips out and then sinks into feelings of guilt, so that you even need to comfort them (after they rudely challenged you). Understandably, this can lead to rejection, which has nothing to do with mobbing, but with "action and reaction".

What can I say: as an ADHDer it might be a good idea, not only to expect understanding from the non-ADHDers, but also be understanding of their situation myself.

And of course, mobbing in the original sense as groundless harassment unfortunately exists in this world.

6.3   Suggested Solutions: Preventing Negative Hyperfocus (Negative Tunnel Vision)

6.3.1   Percentage of Own Self-Regulation

The most important thing to prevent negative hyperfocus is firstly to become as familiar as possible with how it functions in ADHD, and secondly, to practise handling negative hyperfocus repeatedly. "Again and again"—but not all the time.

It's important to be clear that if you have been able to reduce the frequency and intensity of such experiences, you have achieved a lot. No one can do this completely. But it makes a decisive difference whether you feel attacked several times a day, think you have to defend yourself and doubt your own worth, or whether you feel that way once a week. In the first case, life is a torment, with almost paranoid sensations. In the second, you develop a rather relaxed sense of self-confidence, despite an occasional dip.

The difference is reflected in your quality of life, a greater sense of satisfaction and more calmness. Less anger, less loss of energy and time, less self-doubt and bitterness. Of course, the difference is also reflected in the fact that there are fewer unnecessary conflicts arising from misunderstandings. Both workplace and private relationships suffer less damage.

6.3.2   Percentage of Pharmaceutically Supported Self-Regulation

In addition to knowledge and practice, stimulants can also help reduce negative hyperfocus from being easily triggered in ADHD. This must always be discussed individually with those treating the patient. It is crucial to remember that the aforementioned effect only occurs during the time when the drug actually has an effective level in the blood. There are substantial individual differences, both in the size and the duration of the drug level required.

The length of time that the stimulants are effective is often shorter than noted in the manufacturer's instructions, especially in the case of the sustained-release drugs. The time from mid-afternoon to early evening, a period during which everyone is more sensitive owing to normal fatigue, is often when the drugs provide an insufficient level of coverage. Under certain circumstances, it may make sense to adjust the medication accordingly, always in consultation with your physician. It is definitely important to keep a particularly good eye on "yourself" during this period. In general, it's very important to observe the effects of the medication carefully and discuss the observations with your doctor.

6.4   Suggested Solutions: What Do I Do if I Get into Negative Hyperfocus?

6.4.1   First Step: Learn to Recognise Negative Hyperfocus Yourself

The most important thing:

- At as early stage as possible, **I**
- must be capable of **noticing and determining** myself,
- **that** I am in negative hyperfocus
  = *conditio sine qua non* (a necessary condition)

If we cannot recognise this *ourselves*, nothing is going to work, or we're not going to be able to do anything—yes, we can't do anything because we have no reason to.

In order to better understand this, it is worthwhile thinking ourselves deliberately into the condition of negative hyperfocus. Or even better, feeling our way into it:

> *If I only notice that my boss has said something about a fundamental mistake, then I am just convinced that I now realise MORE CLEARLY THAN EVER that he is ONLY EVER so critical of ME, and makes COMPLETELY impossible demands, while he himself NEVER complies with these conditions, and ALSO does NOT make these demands from my colleague. ONLY from ME. He NEVER acknowledges my performance, I can see that ABSOLUTELY CLEARLY NOW!… and so on.*

In this state, no one spontaneously comes up with the idea that they have tunnel vision and that they are perceiving something in a distorted way.

And in this condition, it usually doesn't help if someone tells you that you are in negative hyperfocus. Especially if they are right and point out that the boss said that you had never ever made a fundamental mistake...

So, the first thing to do is to find a way to identify this condition yourself.

You can train a reflex for this purpose, a reflex that uses a typical and always present "symptom" of any negative hyperfocus as a trigger stimulus:

> *Always when I have a particularly strong reaction to something, a particularly negative feeling, then <u>my knee-jerk reaction is to ask the following question: "could it be that I am in negative hyperfocus?"</u>*

Be careful:

It's not a good idea to believe that having a strong reaction to something is always evidence of negative hyperfocus.

The procedure of "asking yourself a question" is important for two reasons:

1. Having a very intense reaction can actually be appropriate once, and does not necessarily have to be caused by tunnel vision. Everyone is aware of this deep down, including every ADHDer. Thus, if they were to automatically attribute tunnel vision to every intense reaction, then no normal ADHDer would take the procedure seriously—and consequently miss the first and decisive step towards resolving the possible existence of negative hyperfocus.
2. By asking yourself a question, you position yourself a little bit outside yourself. This little bit (nothing more!) is usually also possible when you are in hyperfocus. This little bit of distance is just enough to allow you to determine the presence of a restricted view. And it happens while you are still in it. My experiences in recent years have fortunately shown that almost every ADHDer, if they make an effort, can quickly and successfully become an accomplished self-diagnostician in terms of negative hyperfocus.

6.4.2   Second Step: Actively Get Out or Sit It Out?

If you have made the self-diagnosis of negative hyperfocus you need to answer a second question:

Do I want to actively come out of the tunnel vision or just sit it out?

Any negative hyperfocus will eventually dissolve on its own. Of course, you have the freedom not to fight it actively, but simply to wait. This is not necessarily pleasant, but it's your own freedom of choice and can sometimes be useful: if I get into tunnel vision shortly before midnight, but it has been my experience that it does not disturb my sleep and is gone in the morning, then it is not worth much effort. And sometimes you may want to wallow in such a narrow swamp like this, in a mood of rightfulness and reproach. This is part of your freedom—as long as you are prepared to take the consequences.

6.4.3   Third Step: Methods to Get Out of Negative Hyperfocus Actively

If I have decided to take an active approach, I now have to choose the method: *non-specific or specific, or a combination of the two?*

6.4.3.1 Active, Unspecific: Maintaining Cognitive Orientation

Even if negative hyperfocus feels bad and I feel deeply uncertain, tending towards a feeling of being unworthy and incompetent: it makes sense to stick to as clear and simple a focus as possible. In retrospect, we all know that the emotional perception within negative tunnel vision was not realistic but actually catastrophically distorted and had led to catastrophic decisions and actions.

As banal as it may sound and as much as you may resist it:

- In such situations, it simply makes sense to say to yourself: at the moment, I CANNOT rely on my own emotional assessment, of all things.
- Although this does not yet give a differentiated view, it clearly specifies where I am not going, which at least gives you an initial—and essential—point of focus.

The guideline "at the moment I CANNOT rely on my emotional assessment" is difficult to digest, especially for ADHDers. After all, many ADHDers have learned particularly well to assess situations figuratively and emotionally in their coping mechanisms. Such assessments are often correct, but by no means in negative hyperfocus.

Sometimes a comparison with airline pilots helps us to accept this requirement better: It's known that one's instinctive perception of the situation in the air is absolutely unreliable. This can go so far that you are actually in a steep descent, but you are convinced that you are going up. The dangerousness of such misperceptions is obvious. All pilots—even the best ones—are therefore NOT guided by their feelings, but by an instrument called an artificial horizon. Actually, this is an objective horizon, which indicates the real position of the aircraft in space (Fig. 6.1).

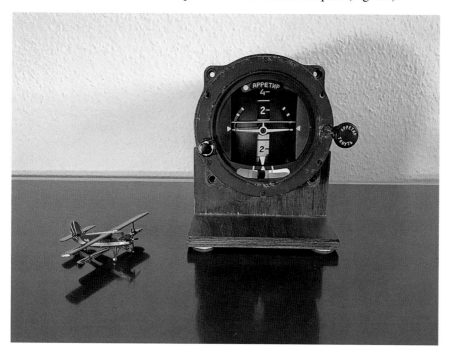

Fig. 6.1 Artificial (objective) horizon: in turbulent situations or in the case of poor visibility (≙ negative hyperfocus), an artificial horizon provides security; flying "by instinct" means that you will crash. Instrument of Antonov An-2 = "tractor of the skies", one of the most reliable aircraft ever built

The equivalent for an ADHDer in negative hyperfocus would be: I do NOT follow my instinctive assessment, but only assess the situation definitively when I am out of the turbulence and fog of negative hyperfocus. I won't decide until then. In the meantime, I am guided by one of my objective reference points, such as "despite all the difficulties, I have made my way again and again".

6.4.3.2 Active Unspecific: Distraction

Distraction—this is advice that you rarely hear from psychiatrists and psychologists. Distraction is usually regarded as a cowardly, shirking evasive manoeuvre by most of my profession. But in negative hyperfocus, distraction or momentary evasion makes perfect sense.

It means nothing more than focussing on something else. In other words: actively leaving the tunnel vision. That's a good move!

Distraction also means seriously realising that a conflict discussion is absolutely pointless as long as you are in negative hyperfocus. The only outcome from this kind of discussion is that the conflict escalates further and a relationship suffers further damage. Regardless of whether this concerns a private or a working relationship.

So, when it comes to a conflict between two people, if there is negative hyperfocus, distraction in the sense of a physical distance is usually required first.

> **Encore**
> The only purpose of this kind of distraction is to leave the tunnel vision. Of course, it should not be a general rejection of discussion. It's just that this should take place at a different time, when everyone is more or less out of the tunnel vision.

There are countless methods that are helpful for distraction. For ADHDers, it is crucial to prepare in advance in a quiet moment which distraction method you will use if you need to. This increases the chance that you will be able to use the technique of distraction successfully.

Distraction Method: **What—How Much—How Long**

In principle, any method of distraction is possible if it works for you as an individual and does not cause additional problems and damage.

- I do not recommend that you distract yourself with alcohol, drugs, brawls, porn, uncontrolled shopping, speeding, devouring food, etc.
- Otherwise, there should be no limits to the imagination for your own distraction methods.

When you have decided on a method, then it's important to determine the scale of the distraction in advance (or at least, to a certain extent). At most, in two variations, one for low-grade hyperfocus, and one for intense hyperfocus. And probably also a minimal variation of distraction, which is practical directly at your workplace.

- If you decide to take a walk as a form of distraction. Then you would go around the block for the small version, for the larger one you would go into the forest for one or two hours.
- Or you decide to "check out" a TV series. Then this would be, for example, one or a maximum of two shorter episodes in the small variation; several episodes in the larger one. But in no case longer than until the time at which, according to experience, you usually fall into a dull, passive mood.
- Examples of minimal variations during work: short toilet visit; short retreat into an "inner exile" with two minutes of immersion in a fantasy story; a short relaxation exercise, or similar.
- The distraction can, as far as the working conditions allow, also lie in alternating with another task, whereby the task triggering the negative hyperfocus is then resumed the following day.

I would like to emphasise again that determining the type and extent of distraction *in advance* is enormously important. In an emergency, you can resort to your choice of distraction automatically, without having to think about it. This gives you an opportunity to find focus, even if you are in tunnel vision mode, and actually to be able to free yourself from it.

6.4.3.3   Active Unspecific: Restoring Emotional Orientation (Contact to a Sense of Your Own Worth)

In negative hyperfocus, ultimately, the contact with your own sense of self-worth is torn away. The most direct way out of negative hyperfocus is to restore contact to your sense of self-worth—the perception of self-worth. It is not the easiest way, but it can be learned and can save a lot of suffering.

Important: it is not only about retrieving your self-worth cognitively (knowledge related to reality), but also perceiving your self-worth emotionally again (feeling related to reality).

In no case should it be a matter of convincing yourself of an illusory worth.

For this purpose, the method of the internal treasure chest "My Treasured Self" has proven to be useful.

The Short Version to Internalise the Idea

In a quiet moment you collect a few (!) personal characteristics, skills or achievements in this imaginary internal treasure chest from various areas which you can use to *feel* your self-worth when you think about it. If you get into negative hyperfocus, and want to actively fight your way out again, you retrieve these areas with the associated (inspired) feeling. This puts you in touch with your own sense of self-worth again, and thus expands your focus. The hyperfocus can resolve more quickly.

Detailed Version to Understand the Implementation of the Idea

The image of an internal treasure box with the name "MY TREASURED SELF" is deliberately chosen suggestively. The treasured treasure of the EGO-self. As a suggestive positive image, it has the best chance of breaking through the constricting perceptual barrier during negative hyperfocus. However, the values collected in it must correspond to reality. The suggestion should only serve as a means to achieve contact with your real worth.

How Much, and Why Only a Few Things?

In this little box, which is supposed to represent the best of yourself, you place only a few characteristics, skills or achievements of yours that you are proud of.

Some ADHDers feel resigned at first, that there is nothing, or hardly anything, that is worth it. In conversation, we can usually find a lot of things. Typically for ADHD, one's own successes, positive qualities and expertise are not part of the active memory treasure, but can be activated (see also Sect. 7.1).

Even if, in the end, numerous such values are identified: it is important that you only choose a few for this TREASURED SELF—a maximum of six treasures. The reason lies, quite tritely, in the way ADHD works. If you get into tunnel vision (having had your worth allegedly called into question), and have to choose between 57 treasures on which you could focus, this would trigger countless thought trees. You would quickly lose track, and be unable to decide which method you should use to support yourself. In other words, even if you had a filled treasure chest the size of Scrooge McDuck's, it would be no help at all, because you would then be faced with an agony of choice.

It's different when you look at a neatly organised treasure chest with six compartments. Here your choice is not prevented by overthinking. What's more, owing to the small number of goods stored in it, each one has more weight on its own, and can be emotionally recalled more easily.

What and How to Distribute?

Actually, it doesn't matter what kind of treasures you choose. The most important thing is—when you think about it—that you are able to *feel* your own value. This is the only thing that counts. Basically, there are a few classic categories:

- Officially recognised achievements:
    e.g. completion of a vocational training course; good performance in a certain task; courageous commitment in a dangerous situation; sporting or political success; had a reasonable career despite setbacks; received an award.
- Officially irrelevant, but achievements that are important to me:
    For example, I scored a wonderful goal in 3rd grade; hardly anyone drives around bends in the car with as beautiful a curve as me; and much more.
- Things I can't do anything about:
    e.g. I have beautiful green eyes; proud of my family of origin; my talents; etc.

- Personality traits:

  e.g. loyalty without submissiveness; integrity; courage; tolerance (well, most of the time) with simultaneous adherence to principles; reliability (in principle, even if often too late); kindness; perseverance; etc.
- Intimate subjective self-assessments that I would never tell anyone about (I don't have to either):

  e.g. no one is as tender as me; sometimes I kiss really well; the night with XX I was a great lover; I'm actually cool and intelligent; etc.
- Ironic:

  e.g. I have the most beautiful teeth, although they are actually dentures – but I can live with it (said by a person who had never brushed his teeth, and already needed false teeth at the age of 30).

  Ironic treasures only work if the more important part is something positive (here: I forgave myself and accepted my previous mistakes, but did not repress them).

The selected treasures should not all come from the same area. So not all from your profession, sport, or personal relationships, etc. The reason is obvious: if only sports achievements are used for your perception of self-worth, it will be difficult to quickly call up a new treasure if you suddenly have to give up sporting activity owing to an injury.

What to Bear in Mind and How to Practise?

It's not about finding the most amazing, achievements or personality traits in yourself. Rather, it's about being able to feel your own worth in those selected. It's a good idea to practise calling up this feeling every now and then in quiet moments.

Feelings always have a physically perceptible component. It's about calling up this component, the physical empathy. For example, the pleasant feeling of warmth in the stomach, paired with a light but clear mind, combined with the self-evident, physical security that comes from contact with one's own potential. This is an example of a corresponding physical perception. It can manifest itself in various ways, depending on the person.

If we are able to call up this sense of our own worth in quiet moments, we can start to practise using it in hyperfocussed situations. You should not forget: no matter what you learn in life, you always start with simple situations. You learn skiing on the "beginner slopes", not on the Lauberhorn Mountain. And: falling on your bum from time to time is normal, and shouldn't discourage you.

> **Encore**
> You can of course create an actual treasure chest for yourself (see Fig. 6.2). This makes it easier to call up the corresponding knowledge and feeling, since you are able to see and touch the box and its contents.

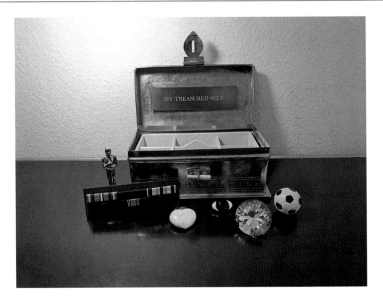

Fig. 6.2 My treasured self: model of an internal treasure chest—a way to access the perception of one's own values more easily

Putting It "Into Action"

If, in a negative hyperfocus situation, you are able to recall your sense of self-worth, this means that you have already taken a first step to expanding your restricted focus—your field of vision. You will be able to recognise the situation that triggered the hyperfocus again in the overall scheme of things—at least partly. As a result, your own assessments, reactive feelings and reactive actions align with the true situation.

> **Encore**
> A brief overview of self-management in negative hyperfocus:
>
> - Learn to notice yourself when you have fallen into negative hyperfocus.
> - Distract yourself where it makes sense and is possible (shift your mental point of focus).
> - Restore contact to your sense of self-worth (expanding the focus on yourself as a whole person).
> - Classify the triggering situation in the overall scheme of things (expand the focus to the overall context in which the current situation takes place).

References

Claus D, Aust-Claus E, Hammer PM. Das A.D.S-Erwachsenen-Buch. Ratingen: Oberstebrink Verlag; 2005.

Lachenmeier H. Selbstwertwahrnehmung bei ADHS Erwachsener. Swiss Arch Neurol Psychiatry. 2014;165(2):47–53.

Neuhaus C. Lass mich, doch verlass mich nicht. Munich: Deutscher Taschenbuchverlag; 2005.

The Self-Worth Issue

7

We have discussed the characteristics of ADHD and their influence on the world of work in various constellations. It is noticeable that there is almost always a distortion in the perception of one's own worth (Solden 2002).

Almost always—but not all the time!

Of course, not every ADHDer has problems in this regard. Even where an ADHDer has difficulties with their perception of self-worth, it doesn't have to stay that way. These difficulties are consequences of ADHD, in other words they are not at all hereditary (Neuhaus 2003). The three main factors for a negative self-image in ADHD are:

- Less automatic pre-filtering of information, a resulting inability to "get the big picture" and, as a result, misinterpretations about oneself and the environment.
- The mechanism of negative hyperfocus, and its ability to wear people down over time, including negative misinterpretations about oneself and the environment.
- Uncomprehending and negative feedback from one's environment, which ADHDers experience significantly more often in the course of growing up than non-ADHDers.

Under these conditions, small events can sometime have a devastating effect. In a best-case scenario, this devastating effect can be prevented or subsequently reduced with little effort (Beerwerth 2007).

7.1 Career Sabotage: ADHD-Specific Self-Perception Falsification

As we have seen several times now, ADHD plays a major role in how a professional career proceeds. It is best to take this genetic condition into account as soberly as possible, using common sense and logical thinking.

© The Author(s), under exclusive license to Springer Nature
Switzerland AG 2023
H. Lachenmeier, *ADHD and Success at Work*,
https://doi.org/10.1007/978-3-031-13437-1_7

- On the one hand, it should not be underestimated how much ADHD can get in the way and slow us down.
- On the other hand, our own potential as ADHDers should not be underestimated either.

Time and again I have observed that a surprisingly number of capable and bright ADHDers are excessively reserved in their professional careers. Despite good qualifications, they reject career paths because they doubt their own ability. The application for a management position is hastily withdrawn in favour of an allegedly better colleague. Healthy ambition and normal competitive behaviour are shunned needlessly.

Case Study 12
The Top Surgent Who Found Career Offers Embarrassing
A few years ago, I had a young surgeon, Zdenka, as a patient. She had completed her training as a specialist in the best university hospitals, had also participated in research projects and in between worked for Médecins sans frontières in war zones for almost a year. She had recently completed her certification as a specialist with flying colours. Now she had been offered a post-doctoral position. Such positions are rarely offered; a certain amount of assertiveness, if not elbowing, is usually necessary to get started in a university career. At the same time, Zdenka also received an offer from a renowned private hospital, financially extremely rewarding.

Of course, she was delighted. But immediately, agonising self-doubt set in. Zdenka was no longer sure whether her professional competence was really that good. Actually, she saw herself more in the middle. What if it turned out that she wasn't that good, because after all, she herself suspected that she had simply been lucky so far. She even considered whether she had been offered the positions by mistake.

I asked Zdenka why she thought she had received two top offers from different institutions. Almost indignantly, she said that was the embarrassing thing—now she would certainly be accused of being arrogant! It didn't occur to her at all that it could also mean—and really did mean—that she was an outstanding young doctor. This visibly astonished her.

It's important not to be fooled: even successful and outwardly calm and self-confident ADHDers can also have such insecurities, of all genders.

As an ADHDer, it is important to be aware of these possible distortions. As a general rule:

- Not only do ADHDers underestimate their own potential
- But they also overestimate that of other people

Unless the other people have proved to be unreliable or not very capable in an obvious and extreme way. In this case, these people are totally rejected by the ADHDer.

It is understandable that under such distortions ("self-perception falsification"), ADHDers tend not to pursue goals that they may want achieve and for which they might have the skills, because they are not aware of their qualities. Not daring to do things that are possible.

• If a colleague is given precedence during a promotion, and over time he proves to be capable, but no more than that, a difficult dynamic sets in.
  The ADHDer forgets that he backed down previously, the responsibility is instead shifted to the outside. The person concerned feels underappreciated and ignored by his superiors. This inevitably leads to tensions in the employment relationship.
• And of course, when it comes to collaborating with others, it is even more unhelpful if an employee who is assessed as moderately competent is rejected as incompetent for all time, just because he slipped up somewhat badly on one occasion.

If you are aware of these possible distortions, and know how they come about, you can successfully prevent them from having a negative influence.

7.1.1   Development of ADHD-Specific Self-Perception Falsification

When ADHDers think about something or someone, their less automatic weighting of thoughts leads to a greater number of branched thoughts than in non-ADHDers. It's impossible to go over these countless thoughts in your mind conclusively, meaning that you get stuck in preliminary, possible assessments (Fig. 7.1).

Experience has shown that the way in which ADHDers deal with these kinds of preliminary positive or negative assessments is primarily dependent on whether these assessments affect themselves or someone else.

• When evaluating fellow human beings, the motto usually is: don't be unfair to them. This means that from the preliminary assessments, the person's possible positive characteristics are already calculated to be on the safe side, while the possible negative ones are not yet taken into account.

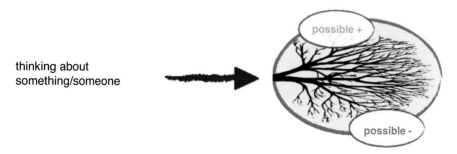

Fig. 7.1 In the case of unchecked thought trees, the evaluations are more often tentative rather than definitive

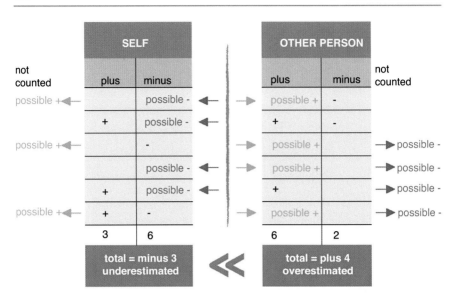

Fig. 7.2 ADHD-specific "self-perception falsification" to the detriment of one's self-worth

- When evaluating oneself, it's possible to observe the exact reverse of this process. The tentatively positive areas are left out as a precaution; the possibly negative ones are sometimes blamed on yourself: it would be so embarrassing if it turned out that you are not so good after all (Fig. 7.2).

In this way, we tend to overestimate "the other person", while at the same time underestimating ourselves. Together, this can lead to a significant distortion of real skills ratios.

It's not surprising that we can quickly lose faith in our own chance, even in very normal competitive situations, as long as we do not know how this (mis-)perception came about.

Other factors that can intensify a lack of self-worth in a worst-case scenario:

- In fields that ADHDers have worked on in detail, they have not merely a vague overview of the field. Rather, they have far-reaching knowledge, they know their way around—they know this field like the back of their hands, as the saying goes. However, very few are aware of this and ADHDers are convinced that these skills are absolutely self-evident—almost every child knows them.
- The same applies to the highly trained ability of many ADHDers to extrapolate (see Sect. 5.4.2). It refers to the ability to derive the sum of things from fragmentary information, with a high success rate. Again, very few ADHDers are aware of their quality in this regard, and assume that every reasonably intelligent person can do the same.

Lack of awareness of these qualities leads ADHDers to significantly underestimate their personal abilities. Naturally they tend to overlook their own advantages against those of competitors as well as the real opportunities against them. It's a pity!

Caution: for the sake of completeness, I would like to mention at this point that not all ADHDers automatically have these skills. In the same way that not all ADHDers exhibit all the possible negative symptoms of the condition.

7.1.2   Suggested Solutions for ADHD-Specific Self-Perception Falsification (Self-Underestimation)

7.1.2.1 Compare Yourself Consciously with Others!

Psychiatrists, psychologists, philosophers and theologians like to spread the alleged wisdom that comparing yourself with others can only make you miserable.

This is not entirely true.

Basically, we humans would not be able to survive without the ability to compare and contrast. We should rejoice in this ability. Without it, we wouldn't exist. And if it were not sufficiently available to us, then we would suffer considerably more in our (ADHD) life.

Of course, one can take comparisons too far. Naturally it's not helpful if people believe that they are only good enough if they are the best, the greatest, the wealthiest, etc. in everything.

Whether we have ADHD or not, we can hardly do anything sensible, either alone or in partnership with others, without comparisons. Without the ability to compare things, we cannot make a meaningful choice; relationships would be largely random and hardly engaging. Our own insecurity would be huge, as we would have no tool to decide between positive and negative; between capable and incapable; friendly or hostile and so on. Most people do this reality check automatically, without even being aware of it.

In ADHDers, on the other hand, this comparison is often not completed owing to the sprawling trains of thought they can lose themselves in, leading to the self-perception falsification described above.

If the consequences of this are to be prevented, comparison with others is definitely recommended. However, this should be done consciously, systematically and time and again from afresh. It is important to keep your own strengths and weaknesses in mind and to weigh them up against those of others in a neutral-objective way.

– The goal and purpose is that you recognise and remain aware of the position of your specialist competences, team abilities and leadership skills in the group. The comparison serves to help your own orientation. Whether it's in your department, occupational group, age group or among your group of employees or self-employed professionals and so on.

– Comparison: a hiker periodically compares his surroundings in confusing terrain with his map, to make sure that he is travelling in the right direction. That gives him peace of mind. Through periodic adjustment, he notices if he deviates from the path at an early stage, which allows him to correct his route in time. In this way, the hike—or the career path—can be taken much more calmly and confidently.

– The comparison described here realistically lifts the lid on your own potential, makes it easier to see which tasks you can cope with, prevents you missing the right time to make a career move, as well as losing time and energy owing to a need to change your route at a late stage.

Encore
To avoid misunderstandings: this kind of comparison has absolutely nothing to do with exaggerated competitive behaviour, with excessive striving for power; in short, with pathological narcissism. We are not talking about destructive victory or annihilation in defeat here.

And it also has nothing to do with submissive over-adaptation to your environment.

It's all about your own orientation in order to get a realistic assessment of yourself vis-à-vis your environment. It's about having a certainty about the real situation.

What you do with this assessment—either hold back and learn, plunge into a competitive struggle, try to adapt, go your own way unswervingly, assert yourself— is a different decision. A decision which can then be made with greater freedom.

7.1.2.2 My External Sensor Is a Person I Trust

In contrast to making a general comparison between yourself and others, this suggested solution is about using a trusted person as a designated sensor in your environment. A sensor where you can get feedback. The person acts as a point of reference and focus for any insecurity that may emerge, to compare your own estimation with that of a reliable third party.

It can be a colleague within your business or a friend from outside with whom you make this arrangement. The following is crucial, however:

- You know this person to be trustworthy and honest towards you. You can rely on receiving fair but honest feedback, both positive and negative.
- You have made a conscious decision to be ready to obtain this feedback, to examine it without any reservations, but also to acknowledge it as a point of focus. By "acknowledge" I do not mean to suggest that you cannot question the feedback. But that you acknowledge that your sensor, whom you trust in principle, has made their assessment to the best of their knowledge and conscience.

You should discuss the procedure with your sensor in a spirit of openness. Otherwise, you will give your external sensor the impression that you are "fishing for compliments" and that you show a lack of independence.

The sensor can be used in various constellations: when assessing a situation, the behaviour of an employee or one's own performance.

Once you have made an *initial assessment* as an ADHDer, an agonising number of possibilities come to mind, all of which could or should be examined and taken into account. Although you regard your assessment as *probably sufficient*, these possibilities sometimes trigger *uncertainty*.

Your external sensor is intended for precisely this situation. If the feedback from your sensor corresponds to your own assessment, your ADHD uncertainty is sufficiently covered and allows you to continue work without delay. If not, it can still be clarified further.

Experience has shown that in the situations in which an external sensor can be used, positive feedback is usually justified. As you can see, you can gain a lot of security when an external person acts as a sensor, and you save both time and energy.

7.1.2.3 Unnecessary Fear: Reality Doesn't Make You Arrogant

When discussing ADHD-specific self-perception falsification and how to overcome it, many of my patients express a fear of becoming arrogant.

In over 20 years of practicing, I have not observed this once; in fact, the opposite tends to be true. The increase in security through a clear perception of one's own qualities—also in comparison with others—creates more calmness, which protects you from becoming arrogant.

By way of explanation:

As long as we are trapped in the emotional rollercoaster of experiencing our own ability, insecurity and agonising self-doubt, we hardly dare to use our qualities to the full. There is no success, but there is plenty of frustration. Especially when we feel our full potential in special moments now and again. Then we feel misunderstood, overlooked and exploited. We distrust all those who are successful. We are confused and angry.

From this uncertainty and bitter anger comes the danger of being aggressively arrogant with the people who surround us.

On the other hand, if we perceive our qualities, use them, assert ourselves constructively, achieve goals and receive appropriate recognition, we feel neither misunderstood nor cheated, neither insecure nor angry, but satisfied and secure.

Then there is no reason to compensate for our frustration by being arrogant. Rather, it will be enriching to meet people who are more competent than ourselves.

7.2 "One-Two-Three-Too Much" or the Mount Everest Syndrome

At the beginning of this chapter on the issue of self-worth, I mentioned that a small event can have a devastating effect. The story below is typical of this kind of small event, which could have very nearly led to greater difficulties. It's a story which teaches us a lot about ADHD and the world of work.

Case Study 13: Part One

The Extreme Sportsman Who Suddenly Took a Lump of Soil for Mount Everest

This is the story of Eric, who was in his mid-40s. He had completed a commercial apprenticeship but did not find it very interesting. He often turned up late for work and was unreliable. After narrowly passing his final apprenticeship exam, he travelled around the world as a backpacker. At first he liked being completely unattached and not subject to any constraints. Spontaneously, or rather impulsively, he followed his changing ideas. When money was tight, he looked for odd jobs. He appeared to be carefree, but didn't quite know what he wanted in life. Eric lived in New Zealand for almost a year, where he worked part-time for a small freight forwarding company. He spent the rest of the time doing Whitewater kayaking, during which time he met his future wife, who had travelled to New Zealand for a kayaking holiday.

They fell in love. Eric returned to Switzerland with her, they wanted to start a family. He soon found a job at an insurance company. One year later, their first child was born.

The new role as a proud husband and father gave Eric a clear direction. It was a task that was important to him. Not unusually for ADHDers, he therefore suddenly showed more reliability and sense of duty for his family than expected. Recently, he endured the rules at work almost without any problems. Every morning, he briefly discussed the upcoming tasks with the boss and completed them on time. Everyone was satisfied.

Until his boss—a calm, quiet man—retired.

The new boss was also an affable man, but with a completely different working style. He appreciated the constant contact with his staff. The morning meetings became short, but he brought Eric each new order personally to the office several times a day. Increasingly, Eric felt overwhelmed at work.

After a short time, the following course of events took place: on the first visit from the boss, Eric accepted the order in a friendly manner with "got it" and even joined in with the boss's chit-chat. At the second and third visit, he became short-tempered, sometimes even grumpy. By the fourth or fifth visit of the boss at the latest, he was swearing to himself under his breath. Sometimes he would explode and complain reproachfully about the ever-increasing work, "and anyway...!"

Every time he exploded like this, he felt bad in several ways. In principle, he acknowledged his boss as a decent, even friendly superior. Eric was ashamed of his uncontrolled behaviour. Moreover, he increasingly doubted his suitability for the job, was afraid of losing the job, of not being good enough as a husband and father and of not leading a worthy life at all.

The last part of the above story illustrates what is described under Sect. 6.2 as the first and second waves of negative hyperfocus. In the first wave: the outbursts towards the boss; in the second: feelings of guilt and self-accusation.

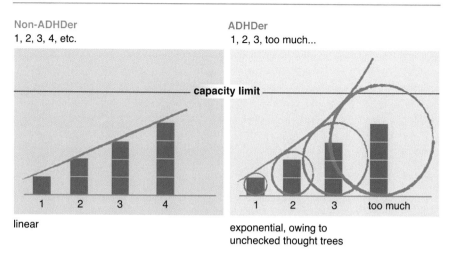

Fig. 7.3 One-two-three-too much

The pattern described in the above case is very common in a similar form among ADHDers. Both in their working and private lives. To put it in a nutshell, the rule of thumb is: ADHDers do not count 1-2-3-4-etc., but 1-2-3-too much (see Fig. 7.3).

- Non-ADHDers simply add each new task to the to-do list. This results in a somewhat linear load curve.
- In contrast, every additional task triggers an unchecked thought tree in the ADHDer, including a connection to all tasks already on the to-do list. This results in an exponentially increasing load curve.
- The load limit is approximately the same for both, but is reached faster by the above-described processes in ADHD.

7.2.1 Suggested Solutions for the Mount Everest Syndrome

Important: the Mount Everest syndrome, the "too much" can be prevented, at least partially. In any case, it is possible to learn to cope with it, to suffer less collateral damage, but especially to avoid misconceptions such as being convinced of your inferiority. To do this, let's continue following the story of the Whitewater canoeist that I started above:

Case Study 13: Part Two

The Extreme Sportsman Who Suddenly Took a Lump of Soil for Mount Everest

How did it come to the alleged overload?

After asking for precise details, it turned out that his volume of work with the new boss had not actually increased at all. It was the exactly the same as before. Subjectively, however, it seemed to Eric that his workload was constantly increasing. This realisation astonished Eric, and aroused his curiosity to get to the bottom of the cause of his subjectively different experience.

It soon became clear what was increasingly stressing him. The new boss came to his office several times a day to bring a new order. Every further order placement triggered an unrestrained, unfiltered thought tree for Eric, an ADHDer—they were conscious and subliminal associations. These had to be compared with the previously received orders, which caused the number of connections to increase exponentially with each new order.

While non-ADHDers can respond with "make a note of it, save it, continue from where you were" with each new order, ADHDers have to check all these newly initiated connections. So, each receipt of an order means a significant, additional use of the computing power of the brain.

- As a result, the small hill of the usual tasks begins to look like Mount Everest: almost or totally impossible to cope with. Not even an extreme athlete could climb Mount Everest every day. They would be compelled to give up.
- Furthermore, the logically longer-lasting distraction makes it more difficult to find your thread again and continue with the previously started task. This is additionally frustrating.

This **purely quantitative overload due to the thought trees triggered several times a day**, was the source of his problem. Eric felt completely overwhelmed, doubted his worth, did not think he was good enough. The focus of the negative hyperfocus, the first wave, was aggressive defence. Subsequently, by recognising the overreaction, the second wave was filled with regret, shame and an **alleged sense of inferiority**.

I would like to emphasise again: the overload was caused by the repeated classification of the newly arrived tasks, not any additional tasks! At no time was the overload due to the type and amount of work. Eric was neither overwhelmed nor overburdened by the actual work. As soon as Eric was able to recognise this, he became aware of his qualities, his worth—not only cognitively but also emotionally.

This allowed him to confidently and respectfully talk with his boss. He explained the course of events as a personality trait, without actually naming the potentially hot topic of "ADHD" for the time being. On this basis, he asked the boss to bring the orders collected as far as possible only once or twice a day. As it was even more convenient for him, he suggested picking up the orders himself from the boss twice a day.

Since Eric initiated the conversation, was able to explain his personality trait in a plausible way, and the boss reacted to it reasonably, the result was a classic win-win situation.

- Eric became more aware of his competence again, felt more confident, was less stressed and more relaxed both in at work and at home.
- The boss no longer had any reason to doubt his employee's qualifications and ability to work in a team.

As is so often the case with ADHD difficulties, the solution lies in understanding the course of events.

7.2.1.1 Stopping Misperception of an Alleged Sense of Inferiority
If we understand that the impression of our own overload is based neither on the type nor the quantity of tasks involved, but on the additional "computational work", then we can overcome the misperception of alleged inferiority. At first mainly cognitively, but with increasing understanding, also emotionally.

7.2.1.2 Simple Tactics to Prevent Trigger Situations
- Organisationally, depending on the nature and structure of the work, it's worthwhile looking for opportunities that follow the **rule of thumb**: "only one order is placed, for example, per half-day or day; the number and scope of the orders then only play a secondary role".
  Or correspondingly if you are a manager with ADHD: if it is not absolutely urgent, the employees can only contact you for questions at defined time windows.
- And just as important: if the principle of "1-2-3-too much" applies to ADHD, then this also applies in the opposite direction! In other words "too much-3-2-1".
  In other words: if you feel overloaded, you can sometimes find and feel an overview by completing a single, minor task. The reduction by one task leads to an exponential *decrease* of the possible associations and thus the impression of an alleged overload.
  Rule of thumb: "when I feel overloaded, I immediately do a small task that does not necessarily have to be important. The chances are good that I will be able to get an overview again afterwards".
- For self-orientation, the **rule of thumb**: "when I see Mount Everest in front of me in my everyday life and want to give up, it's probably just a small hill. It would be better to take a closer look first".

Of course, sometimes there really is "too much" at work, but that's another story.

7.3   My Personal No-Goes

7.3.1   What Am I Sure I Won't Do, Even if I Could?

Be careful! It's easy to misunderstand this subchapter. Naturally I don't want you *not* to aim to improve how you deal with your ADHD. In no case should you just resign yourself to thinking something along the lines of, "ADHDers just can't do that..." And certainly, you should not use ADHD as an excuse.

BUT: sometimes there are things which are enormously difficult for ADHDers, *although* they would technically have the ability to do them. So enormously difficult that the "enormously difficult" is not putting it strongly enough. And that's just the way it is. Things that you ultimately know you won't get done—no-goes.

These can be very different things for different people.

Case Study 14
The Psychiatrist Who Was Allergic to Accounting
I know, for example, that I am good at keeping accounts. Compelled to do this by the path I took in life, I have mastered it many times, both for associations for which I worked, when organising international congresses, or in my practice.

It's just that, ever since I had to keep the milk book accounts (a simple income/expenditure calculation) of the class cash register when I was at school, this has been a horror for me. As soon as I am confronted with such a task, I feel absolutely incapable. I almost physically feel an almost insurmountable wall of thick reinforced concrete before me. My stomach becomes queasy, my head buzzes and is empty, dull. I will spare you the description of the remaining symptoms. Many of you probably know them better than you would wish.

As mentioned: compelled by my path in life, I have mastered such tasks. But it always took a huge amount of energy. Incomprehensibly huge in the eyes of others—and formerly incomprehensible to me too.

Because of my lack of understanding, I fatally assumed that I should be able to casually perform these kinds of tasks. This repeatedly led to my energy fizzling out irrationally, to senseless overexertion.

At some point, it seemed less bad to throw away certain receipts for practice expenses than to bother filing them. I kept putting off sending reminders for unpaid bills from patients. In one case until the money could no longer be claimed because the patient had been murdered in the meantime by a husband with whose wife he had been having a romantic affair.

As a result, I came to my senses a little. I realised that it wasn't exactly very clever to attempt to complete my own no-goes with a huge effort on my part but in a rather unsatisfactory way. Today I can rely on an employee who does all this for me.

> Initially I regarded this as an apparent luxury. In reality, the employee saves me nerves, time, energy and a lot of money. Lower fee losses, lower taxes and increased productivity in my core activity significantly exceed the wage and associated costs for the employee. In addition, the collaboration is very pleasant and I would not want to do without it.

The tasks in question do not even have to be extensive, such as preparing a quarterly report on time. It can be small things, such as regularly recording the expenses incurred.

In other words: tasks that are eminently doable; for which one certainly has the requisite knowledge and skills, but an almost immeasurable reluctance to actually get down to them. Nevertheless, it is not uncommon for ADHDers to feel that they have to prove themselves capable of doing exactly these kinds of tasks—which logically leads to **overexertion**.

Or alternatively, the same person may even pretend that these things are not important (**underestimate**). Or you decide to do the task just before finishing work for the day and **procrastinate**. Then you realise that you haven't got enough time and anyway, you're supposed to avoid doing overtime.

Being under the illusion that this kind of task is not one of your duties is also very popular. From this, it easily follows that it is an **unreasonable demand** to be bothered with the task at all. Maybe it's even bullying? As a rule, none of this is true, even if one feels that it is. Usually you suspect this inwardly, but do not want to admit it to yourself.

Why is it so difficult to find a practical way to deal with it? The reason is that there is a misconnection:

If completely banal things are so difficult for me without knowing why, I, as a reasonably thinking person, draw the seemingly logical conclusion that I am stupid.

But only seemingly logical, however, because I do not take the different, functional prerequisite—unknown to me—into consideration. So, the issue is not whether I'm "stupid", but under what conditions I can access my own abilities, which certainly do exist. Most ADHDers are not aware of these backdrops.

Self-doubt and reduced self-confidence are the result. Alternatively, ADHDers may fight back with all their might against the alleged sense of inferiority (see Sect. 3.2.1 and Chap. 6). There is a great temptation to shift the problem away from oneself, to **externalise** it according to the motto: the other person is to blame.

In the short-term, this can make the internal situation more bearable. In the medium- and long-term, it regularly leads to more serious conflicts.

Encore

People manoeuvre themselves into an "offside" position by blaming their company, superiors, colleagues or subordinates for their own shortcomings. Let's be honest, there's actually no excuse for this kind of abusive behaviour—whether you are an ADHDer or not. And the ADHDer doesn't learn to handle their ADHD any better in this way either.

Please note: I don't want to give the impression that all one's problems in life and at work are always only to do with oneself. This is certainly not the case.

In addition to the externalising mechanisms described, **banal cover-up manoeuvres or excuses** are also very common in these kinds of situation.

Of course, when it comes to the topic of one's own no-goes, it's very common to miss deadlines, postpone work or leave things incomplete—this is embarrassing. When asked, it's easy to fall back on improvised excuses and white lies such as, "I did it already but I just can't find it at the moment".

ADHDers often say this with the honest intention of doing it right away. It's just that somehow they forget about it—the task is **dropped like a stone**, you could say. Of course, this can have far-reaching consequences. In no time, one can be burdened with a reputation ranging from "unreliable" to "scheming liar".

Case Study 15
An Honest Liar

A few years ago, a family doctor referred a patient called Valentin to me, who was around 30 years old at the time. The letter of referral indicated that the family doctor had a fine understanding of humanity. It was as concise as it was precise: "Dear colleague, the patient is a casual worker, without training. He has constant problems both at work and with his girlfriend because he does not tell the truth. However, he doesn't seem to be a liar to me, but honest and also intelligent. Maybe you can solve the riddle?"

Exactly what I describe above had occurred in Valentin's case. The in-depth diagnostics revealed ADHD. The more Valentin understood how he functioned, the more he could really perceive and trust in his abilities. He also benefitted from the drug treatment. He no longer saw any need to tell "fibs"—not even to himself. Instead, Valentin dared to do something for the first time in his life.

Soon he began an apprenticeship, successfully completed it, and today works in the administration of a food corporation. The relationship with his girlfriend did not break down; rather, it has improved significantly.

To put it briefly, you should get to know your own "no-goes" well. It's important to identify these areas realistically, but also without a general sense of resignation.

In these areas—and *only* if they really are no-goes—it makes no sense to demand from yourself that they should be overcome by all means. The enormous effort required for this would only be worthwhile in a few cases.

On the other hand, it is essential not to deny under any circumstances your own no-goes, but to include them completely pragmatically in your life with as much common sense as possible.

7.3.2 No-Goes and Professional Self-Employment

An illusion-free classification of one's own no-goes is also crucial, in particular, for ADHDers who strive to be professionally self-employed. Highly qualified, performance-oriented and highly motivated professionals in particular have a high risk of failure (Phillips 2006).

It's easy to delude yourself that you are automatically attracting customers and achieving success with your professional top offer. It's easy to believe that the little bit of administration can be done quickly in the evening by means of smart business software, thereby saving the costs of employing a member of staff.

Unfortunately, this is rarely the case. Some tasks of self-employed working are usually among the no-goes of professionally qualified ADHDers.

Organisation of the business, countless telephone appointments and—even worse—date changes, advertising, acquisition, managing customer contacts, creating cost estimates, ordering materials, cleaning, correspondence, invoicing, incoming payment control, accounting, annual report and tax return are rarely found among the top ten—or the top hundred—of the popular occupations of ADHDers. So, these tasks tend to get forgotten. Everything else seems more important at almost every moment.

In the best case, this will cost time and money. In the worst case, it leads to the ADHDer tragically failing in their self-employed career, despite producing high-quality work.

In this respect, timely acceptance of these no-goes and a pragmatic way of dealing with them is not just a sign of resignation. Rather, it opens up opportunities to delegate the corresponding tasks and structures, which lay the foundation for success in the first place.

7.3.3 Suggested Solutions in Respect of Personal No-Goes

Real no-goes are not as numerous as some suspect. Once you have identified and taken note of your own no-goes, you create the prerequisites for a pragmatic approach to them, and are therefore able to reduce their negative consequences.

By way of distinction:

- My suggested solutions for deciding the relevance of tasks to be completed (see under Sect. 5.2.5) were divided into three parts "zero tolerance", "80/80" and "nice to have". The focus was on the **objective importance** of the task.
- For the no-goes, I propose a similar division into three categories. However, the reference point for the no-goes is your own **subjective feeling** which a task triggers in you. It is completely independent of the importance of a task.

The table below gives you an overview of the subjective feeling, divided into three categories and outlines the basic tactic/way to deal with it/attitude to it (Table 7.1).

Table 7.1 Three-part division: ideal—doable—no-goes

	Activity	Fact	Aim
Ideal activities	– Ability yes – Interest yes – Exciting	Enthusiastically motivated, easy to implement as far as "hard to stop"; positive hyperfocus	– Look for a job with as *high* a proportion of these activities as possible ("niche") – Realistically, remember that this is always only partially possible – In the case of these activities be careful not to do too much or to "flood" other people
Doable, necessary activities	– Ability fundamentally available – Moderate interest – Moderately boring	Can be overcome with reasonable effort; tasks can and must be implemented	– Even with the best job, they always make up a sizeable proportion! – Targeted structuring elements save energy and time – This becomes more possible when you realise that structuring is smart, i.e. not based on an alleged sense of inferiority
No-goes	– Ability in itself exists – Lack of interest; activity triggers complete reluctance – Totally boring	Almost impossible to implement oneself; at the most with disproportionate energy expenditure	– In case of great difficulty: accept that something is one of your own no-goes – Accepting something is not the same as finding something great; it means, being pragmatic – With a level head acknowledge the fact without giving yourself an inferiority complex – Starting from this acceptance find a way not to have to do these kinds of tasks – Consciously and openly, e.g. **delegate or outsource**, in the knowledge that this does not mean you are inferior; rather that this is realistic, resource-saving and clever **Where possible**: – Look for a job with as *low* a proportion of these activities as possible – Sense of reality: having to do a small proportion of tasks that require disproportionate effort is almost unavoidable

References

Beerwerth C. Suche Dir Menschen, die dir guttun. Freiburg: Kreuzverlag Herder; 2007.

Neuhaus C. Das hyperaktive Baby und Kleinkind. Berlin: Urania-Verlag; 2003.

Phillips L. Lawyers with ADHD. GPSolo Magazine; 2006.

Solden S. Journey through adulthood. New York: Walker & Co; 2002.

ADHD Medication and Job

8

When it comes to the drug treatment of ADHD, then methylphenidate (e.g. Ritalin®, Medikinet®, Concerta®) or Dex-methylphenidate (FocalinXR®) and Lis-dexamphetamine (Elvanse®) are the most commonly used drugs. Together with other substances, they form the group known as stimulants, with methylphenidate still being considered the first-choice drug (Müller 2016).

In ADHD, the availability of dopamine and noradrenaline is partially reduced in the brain (see Chap. 3). Stimulants improve the availability of dopamine and noradrenaline. In short, this activates the automatic filter for information and the control of executive functions. This effect is present only as long as the drug is present in the blood, that is, for different lengths of time, depending on the drug, however only for a few hours.

In addition to stimulants, other substances can also be used, in particular those from the group of so-called antidepressants. Ultimately, however, depending on the situation, almost all common psychiatric and various other medicaments can be used.

Be careful:

- Not every ADHDer needs drug therapy
- Not everyone who needs medication needs it all the time

8.1   Purpose of Possible Medication

Medications can *under certain circumstances* play a decisive role in whether you can lead your life with ADHD freely (Luderer et al. 2016). Life also includes your career path. Whether medication is useful or even decisive for someone, and if so which and in what dosage, can only be decided on an individual basis in consultation with the doctor treating you. And: sometimes medications are contraindicated for medical reasons.

The *primary* (medical-psychiatric) purpose of stimulants in ADHD is *not* improved performance. Not even when it's about ADHD and the world of work. It's much more about ensuring that the ADHDer is able to make use of his functions and abilities. The areas in which this is needed depend on the individual concerned. In a professional context, this sometimes concerns organisation and self-organisation at work; sometimes it is more about focussing and sticking with something and sometimes completely different aspects of ADHD.

Of course, this can lead to an increase in performance as a *side effect*.

Sometimes, however, it's about the opposite: the fact that, with the help of medication, you are no longer searching for perfectionism in the "wrong" place can mean that you actually do *less*! You are thereby restricting yourself to your true core activity, meaning that it can be completed in a useful period of time. So the idea is therefore to set boundaries (see also section "Overview of the Relevance of the Tasks to Be Completed").

And sometimes it's not at all about the possible influence of medication on one's performance per se, but about supporting you in your perception of cooperation and the perception of other people in your work environment such as colleagues or clients. In other words, it's about the "human factor", the prevention of misunderstandings and ultimately about helping to shape your range of relationships as the basis of professional work.

8.2   Clarify Possible Career Restrictions!

When choosing a career, it is advisable to clarify at an early stage whether there are legal restrictions for ADHDers who may want to work in a particular profession, especially for those who take stimulants.

Such regulations are not the same in all countries, and they can also change from time to time. Sometimes these are absolute exclusion criteria; sometimes there are insignificant regulations that do not stand in the way of professional practice.

Important: some of these restrictions may not be based on rational justifications. Nevertheless, it is necessary to comply with legal regulations. But also consider that legal regulations are not set in stone. They can be changed through the legislative route, at least in democracies organised by the rule of law.

Encore
In most countries, pilots (not only airline pilots, but also pilots of private sports machines) are not allowed to fly if they are being treated with stimulants. Professional drivers, on the other hand, are also allowed to work if they take stimulants, but receive a coded entry in their driving licence.

8.3   You Should Demand Detailed, Plausible Information About Possible Medication

In the drug treatment of ADHD, the interaction of biochemical-neurological and reactive-psychological factors is important. Similarly, understanding the way ADHD functions is central to appreciating its particular nature. It is necessary to be able to understand medication to a certain extent and at the same time to be able to classify emotionally the effect that drug treatment has and what this means in your own case.

Specifically, it is important to understand the influence of medication on the way your own ADHD functions. Which phenomena may be influenced and what specifically do you need to bear in mind? What effect can you expect? And how long it can last? Only then do the prerequisites for conscious self-observation of changes exist, both in terms of cognitive functions, emotional experience and behaviour.

Often patients are not made aware enough of the fact that they should pay attention to tendencies. For example, that you are only distracted by having a chat twice a day instead of seven times a day. If such quite respectable effects are overlooked, a groundless dose increase often follows, which can sometimes go as far as an overdose.

Discussing the medication takes time, a great deal of time. But it is time that is definitely worth taking (Barkley 2017). As a result, there is less chance that an ADHDer will hastily give up taking the medication, and also less chance of an overdose. As a general rule, it takes at least one and a half hours for a correspondingly detailed, initial medication consultation. This will lay a solid foundation for future treatment.

Encore
In my practice, we use a printed template for the in-depth medication consultation. It's a kind of checklist to ensure that none of the important topics are forgotten.

The patient is given a copy on which he can make additional notes. The categories listed on it are clearly understandable, but the corresponding keywords are deliberately kept incomprehensible. The purpose of this is that there is no distraction from reading the entire sheet during the consultation. I explain this explicitly, but of course I also explain that at the end of the appointment, the keywords will make sense.

Another important goal of the in-depth medication consultation is to make sure that the patient does not make involuntary misconnections. Interestingly, the more intelligent ADHDers in particular seem to have a tendency to subliminally misinterpret medication in the sense that it allegedly proves that they are "damaged goods".

Through closer self-observation and subsequent discussion of personal feedback in subsequent sessions, both the optimal dosage (as much as necessary, but no more than this) and the optimal medicament can be found.

8.4   ADHD Medication on Business Trips

ADHD drugs belonging to the group of substances known as stimulants are subject to the Narcotics Act. I am always amazed at how many patients are not sufficiently informed by their doctors about its importance. In particular, many ADHD patients are not informed that these drugs can only be taken across national borders with a special permit. This applies regardless of whether it is a business or private trip.

> **Encore**
> These certificates are also necessary for some types of painkillers, sedatives and sleeping pills.

The requirements for the permits vary, depending on the country.

In Europe, the form "Certificate for carrying narcotic drugs within the framework of medical treatment—Article 75 of the Schengen Implementing Convention" is usually sufficient; it must be signed by both the doctor and the pharmacist. Unfortunately, it is valid for only 30 days, which is far from practical in everyday professional life.

For other countries, a form signed by a doctor is sometimes sufficient. As a rule, the template of the WHO "Model form of a certificate for the carrying by travellers under treatment of medical preparations containing narcotic drugs and/or psychotropic substances" is used.

For some countries, the WHO form must be stamped in advance by the consulate of the country to be visited.

"Ask your doctor or pharmacist..." also applies here. Many countries provide specific information and corresponding forms on their websites. Sometimes it is also necessary to contact the health authorities of your own country or the consulate of the destination country. Clarifications at consulates can occasionally take a lot of time, in extreme cases up to 3 months.

Plan this aspect of your business trips at an early stage. If you often have to travel to different countries at short notice, it is important that you always keep the permits for the eligible countries up-to-date.

> **Encore**
> Please take these rules seriously. A few years ago, the case of an American woman who worked as an English teacher in Japan went through the press. She had stimulants for her ADHD sent by post, was discovered and spent more than 2 weeks in pre-trial detention. It was only after the ambassador's direct intervention that she was released.

Of course, it is also possible to suspend the medication for the duration of a business trip. However, this is not always recommended. Another possibility is to switch to medications of other substance groups for the duration of a business trip, which have a less specific or less strong effect, but which are not subject to the Narcotics Act.

8.5   Major Occupational Impact of a Common Medication Error

It is often forgotten during stimulant treatment that these drugs are only effective for a relatively short time. This also applies to the so-called prolonged-release preparations which are advertised with the slogan "one per day". Unfortunately, the duration of effectiveness indicated by the pharmaceutical companies is rarely achieved. In a large number of patients, the effect decreases much earlier.

Some doctors and therapists are far too unaware of these circumstances.

As a result, it often happens that a patient who, soon after lunch, once more has the greatest difficulty in organising and concentrating at work, simply receives a higher morning dose because the doctor has not asked enough detailed questions. It is mistakenly assumed that the effect lasts all day.

As a result, an exhausting combination can arise, which can have a particularly devastating effect on working life:

- *Overdose in the First Half of the Day*
  Leading to increased agitation and restlessness, depending on the extent of the overdose or even to a dull, slowed-down state if the overdose is even higher.
- *Underdosing in the Second Half of the Day or from Mid-Afternoon*
  In the best case, the lessening of the drug's effect "only" results in a drop to the patient's untreated state. In a less favourable case, the so-called rebound phenomenon can occur in some patients: the stimulant level drops and there is a lack of energy and mood swings for a certain time (half an hour to several hours). A distressing condition that is exceptionally disadvantageous and frustrating in a work situation.

Encore
To prevent these iatrogenic (= caused by the doctor) medication problems:

If you are a doctor: talk to your patients, describe in detail what they can roughly expect from the medication and when. Question your patients carefully: what exactly, when exactly, for how long exactly, what if not, etc. was observed after taking the medication.

If you are a patient: do not be "patient" for once, ask your doctor, go to him (constructively, friendly) "get on his nerves" until he talks to you in detail. Ask exactly what you should pay attention to, what you might miss if you don't look for it, what to expect more or less, but also what not to expect, how exactly and when you should take what, etc.

So, the treatment of ADHD with drugs is also about observing, reporting, listening, thinking, asking, observing again and so on – both for the doctor and for the patient.

References

Barkley RA. Das grosse Handbuch für Erwachsene mit ADHS. Bern: Hogrefe; 2017.
Luderer M, Bump JM, Sobanski E. Pharmakotherapie der ADHS im Erwachsenenalter. Psychopharmakotherapie. 2016;23:141–50.
Müller TJ. Methylphenidat unverändert der Goldstandard. ADHS bei Erwachsenen spezial, Medical Tribune; 2016.

Transition: Growing Up with ADHD

Adolescence, Career Choice, Education and Further Training

Attention: This chapter is also interesting for adult ADHDers.

- *Some of the mechanisms and coping strategies described here also affect working life.*
- *Thematically appropriate questions on procrastination by eternally doing further training; career planning and other occupational projects are categorised here.*
- *Experience has shown that various earlier, possibly existing difficulties become understandable; or you can find your peace with them in any case.*

Of course, all the issues about ADHD and the world of work do not first arise when an ADHDer starts working life. ADHD can have a major impact on school, career choice and education. It is definitely advantageous to include ADHD in these topics in a down-to-earth way.

These questions are not only of concern to ADHDers themselves, but also to those around them, i.e. parents, friends and also teachers, instructors and lecturers.

I would like to stress again here: it's not about creating a blanket climate of protection, but about incorporating your knowledge about ADHD into your relationships. On this basis, it's easier for you to demand something of someone, and demands made upon you can be coped with more successfully. Let's not forget: most ADHDers get bored quickly if their work doesn't involve challenges. But clearly, meeting the right kind and size of challenge often means walking a tightrope.

© The Author(s), under exclusive license to Springer Nature
Switzerland AG 2023
H. Lachenmeier, *ADHD and Success at Work*,
https://doi.org/10.1007/978-3-031-13437-1_9

9.1   Often Forgotten: What ADHD Also Means in Adolescents

9.1.1   Delayed Maturing of the Brain

Basically, ADHD functions in adolescents and in adults in the same way. Information is less automatically categorised into important and unimportant. The steering and proportioning of executive functions are more dependent on the given situation at that moment.

In addition, there is a delay in brain development during the first 20–25 years, owing to the genetic condition of ADHD (Shaw et al. 2007).

Warning: this is only a delay and by no means an underdevelopment.

The delay is manifested primarily in social and emotional spheres, such as rather childish behaviour. Russel Barcley, one of the most famous American ADHD specialists, states as a rule of thumb that ADHD children and adolescents are on average 3 years younger than their biological age (Barkley 2011).

Alongside the social and emotional lag, ADHDers who have average or good intelligence, can even exhibit a head start over their peers in intellectual fields.

This discrepancy can cause special difficulties in development.

Knowledge about this is useful not only for young people and the people around them. For adults with ADHD, knowing about it can be just as helpful. This often makes it possible to better classify past difficulties in retrospect, to understand oneself better. This is a relief and not infrequently the ADHDer can leave behind any sense of inferiority that may have arisen in this way.

9.1.2   Importance for Social and Emotional Development (Growing Up)

Especially worth mentioning here is the maturing in the area of sexuality and relationships, i.e. puberty and adolescence. This phase of life is difficult, even for non-ADHDers:

- Firstly, the young person is supposed to develop an independent view of the world and life, despite a real and extensive dependence on adults. The inner uncertainty is great and naturally, it is denied. For the time being, the teenager oscillates back and forth between principled total opposition and over-adaptation. In this contradiction, it's impossible to really understand oneself.
- Secondly, there is the additional developmental task of coping with an extremely confusing field of sexual urges and the unknown territory of romantic relationships. Desires and fears form an inner storm. In order to reduce anxiety, the young people in this phase group together with same-sex peers. They take refuge in a chauvinistic attitude—which is to some extent normal for this phase. From this protective peer group, the first attempts are made to approach the coveted-feared prospective romantic partner.

- Ideally, this leads to teenagers gaining a degree of security in dealing with their love life, including the disappointments that are associated with it. Subsequently, age-specific chauvinism should be overcome and more mature development should begin (unfortunately quite a few men *and* women never succeed in doing this).

It is not without reason that this is predominantly experienced as the most difficult phase in everyone's life, although it is often glorified at a later date.

The physical development of puberty is not delayed in ADHD.

I explain the effects of the ADHD condition during this delicate development phase below. Please bear in mind that these descriptions do not apply absolutely. They show typical patterns in an exaggerated way. Things may look completely different in individual cases. There are too many factors influencing our development to be able to describe one exact, typical development. But the exaggerated descriptions can help you to recognise and understand the patterns in your individual situation.

> **Encore**
> Certain patterns are more often observed in boys or girls. But of course, the patterns described in the boys can also occur in the girls, and vice versa.
>
> And naturally the same applies to homosexuals, non-binary, trans people, intersexuals, asexuals, aromantics and others. As a rule, they face even more difficulties during this stage of development.

How do ADHDers deal with the situation of being on an equal footing in terms of physical development yet emotionally and socially a little behind, and intellectually possibly ahead?

9.1.3   ♂—Male ADHDers in Puberty/Adolescence

Two opposite extreme forms:

9.1.3.1 The Rather Extrovert Proactive Daredevil

These ADHDers intuitively grasp the purpose for grouping together in their peer group: everyone wants to go to the girls, but everyone is afraid. This realisation gives a clear orientation. Although not in terms of sexuality and relationships, but within the group. This lowers one's own fear massively.

And it turns the situation into an almost banal test of courage, a stimulus that an ADHDer can hardly resist. He acts first, becomes the peer group leader, so to speak. As part of the test of courage in front of the peer group audience, any rejections by the girls are also accepted. The focus is more on proving one's own daring to the group. If contact does come about, these ADHDers sometimes act out a relationship, possibly without being ready for it.

- In a best-case scenario, they actually overcome the fear of the unknown and soon develop good relationships.
- In the less favourable scenario, they stay searching for the kick, the pattern of the pubertal test of courage, which is about "conquest" and is less conducive to relationships.

9.1.3.2 The Rather Introverted Idealising Romantic

The drive to form a peer group for the purpose of "lowering fear" is not automatic-intuitive in these ADHDers. In their own disorientation (physically equal, emotionally socially a little behind, intellectually ahead), they try to get an overview with their best skill: thinking.

From this perspective, the chauvinist behaviour of the peer group must appear as a completely unacceptable primitiveness.

Consequently, they distance themselves from their own peer group. At the same time, they also begin to feel fear regarding the "battle of the sexes", but remain alone with this. Often the intellectual advantage becomes an obstacle.

- They flee to the cognitive track, on which the behaviour of their peers is completely rejected. The arguments are rationally quite coherent, but are misused for their own anxiety reduction. Extensive and often high-level intellectual activities, even with significantly older people, can obscure puberty or adolescence.
- At the same time, the fear-inducing, impenetrable conglomeration of sexuality and love is idealised. Everything that has to do with it is stylised into an inflated, almost sacred dimension, into something that cannot be fulfilled and cannot be satisfied anyway. Unless, of course, you can prove yourself worthy by some kind of inspired deed. But this probably won't be possible anyway.

    In its grandiosity, this idea may seem meaningful and anxiety-lowering in the short-term, but in the medium-term you are guaranteed to suffer frustration and despair.

It gets bad for these ADHDers when their emotional and social readiness for the corresponding experience catches up. A peer group is then no longer available for them. On the other hand, the fear of sexuality and love is twice as high owing to the romanticising idealising.

- In the best case, a good friend is at your side, or you encounter a sensitive young woman who helps you to overcome the hurdle. However, some people also show special courage and find a way to handle relationships in this situation themselves.
- In the worst case, disorientation and uncertainty will remain for a long time. The persons concerned are enormously ashamed that they only experienced their first sexual contacts or relationships very late, or have not had any at all. Unfortunately, this is far from rare.

    The knowledge of these backgrounds can also be a relief in advanced adulthood and open up new paths.

9.1.4   ♀—Female ADHDers in Puberty/Adolescence

In general, girls are slightly ahead of boys in their development. That's why ADHD girls during puberty are less noticeable than boys. However, there is another reason.

Regardless of the changing role models, the pattern of expecting guys to play an active role in the search for a partner still applies in many layers of society. Regardless of whether this is biologically related or arises mainly from social influences, it offers female teenagers the opportunity not to make the first move themselves, but merely to signal approval or rejection without much effort.

This position may seem enviably comfortable to some male teenagers (with or without ADHD). In fact, a female ADHD teenager can more easily have her first experiences in this way. However, the whole thing also has a downside. It provides a breeding ground for significant ADHD-related accentuated difficulties.

- So, it can be much more difficult for a female ADHD teenager in all her unrestrained-unfiltered associations, thoughts, feelings and urges to clearly notice how far she wants to get involved in a relationship. This doesn't just concern sexual activity, by the way. In the unmanageability of the amount of data, there is an increased risk of overadjustment, compared to female non-ADHDers.
- If this is accompanied by reduced impulse control and the search for the kick, then the probability of unprotected sex is considerable. The incidence of unwanted pregnancies is higher than in non-ADHDers (Østergaard et al. 2017). They often have to deal with the consequences on their own, whether this means an abortion or whether the child is carried to full-term.
- What happens when a female teenager, who is more likely to be passive in a relationship, loses interest in the boy? It is not uncommon for these ADHDers to struggle to gain a clear view of the situation. Do I really not want any him more, or maybe I still do?

  The normal insecurity towards the end of a relationship is clearly emphasised. In addition, there are questions such as "May I even end a relationship?", or "Isn't it unfair if I end a relationship?", or "If I would do everything better, then it would be fine, I'm just not good enough?", or "Can anyone else like me at all?". Due to the ADHD-related flood of data, all these uncertainties are usually much stronger than in non-ADHDers.

  Not infrequently, this leads to the fact that a female ADHD teenager—or later also an adult woman with ADHD—persists for much longer in a relationship that has long since died, or even in one that is characterised by totally destructive patterns.

Encore
The relic of these adolescent hardships in combination with the general functioning of ADHD sometimes shows the following phenomenon in adulthood, in both men and women:

- As an ADHDer, you don't really get an overview of how many of the expectations, wishes and demands of your partner have to be fulfilled. Or how many of the possible "favours of love" that come into your mind would be actually appropriate.
  - **So, you just do "everything".**
- In the same way, the appropriate level of your own claims to "favours of love" from your partner remains unclear.
  - **So, you demand—almost—nothing.**

The consequences of this are devastating:

- Your partner increasingly experiences you as a kind of service provider. This can be very comfortable for your partner, but certainly not attractive.
- The partner, provided that everything is done for him/her, can no longer contribute anything to the relationship and feels that they are useless to you. Nobody wants that.
- The ADHDer feels increasingly exploited. And develops the impression that a love relationship is synonymous with self-abandonment.

Self-abandonment, or giving up on yourself—of course, no normal person wants that.

It's usually only in middle age that another logical conclusion follows from this which, however, is wrong, since it is based on wrong prerequisites. Namely, "I do not want a love relationship at all".

At the end of this subchapter, I would like to repeat: the patterns described here are more common, partly in boys and partly in girls with ADHD. Of course, they can also occur in the opposite sex or any other gender variant. And I would like to repeat again: these behavioural patterns can persist well into adult life.

9.1.5   Significance for School and Education

ADHD can have many implications for school and training that should not be underestimated. Some are specifically mentioned here.

The **discrepancy** between emotional-social developmental delay and sometimes having been intellectually ahead, can cause difficulties in school or training. An almost childish carefree attitude or also an impulsive silliness become gradually less

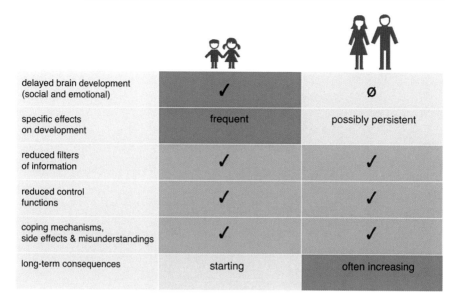

delayed brain development (social and emotional)	✓	Ø
specific effects on development	frequent	possibly persistent
reduced filters of information	✓	✓
reduced control functions	✓	✓
coping mechanisms, side effects & misunderstandings	✓	✓
long-term consequences	starting	often increasing

Fig. 9.1   Comparison of ADHD in childhood/adolescence and adulthood

compatible with educational institutions and the world of work as you approach adulthood. Don't forget that an ADHDer will catch up their underlying delay in brain maturation at a later stage.

However, the basic mechanisms of ADHD remain (see Fig. 9.1). It is worthwhile, however, looking for individual ways on how best to deal with them or how to find better self-regulation at an early stage (Döpfner 2011). The influence of ADHD on the school career of ADHDers depends heavily on their personal **interests**. If they are generally interested in the school subjects and have average intelligence, these ADHDers are much less noticeable than when the subjects bore them.

It is not uncommon to find ADHDers who performed moderately or even poorly at school, but who absolutely blossomed during vocational training. Even in subjects they previously rejected, they achieve top grades. The combination of the positive hyperfocus due to the high interest in the job with the concrete, occupational significance of the subject they used to hate, helps them to concentrate.

Encore
As described above, vocational training chosen because of interest often enables a spontaneous **link between positive hyperfocus and an unloved task**. It's even possible to aim specifically for this kind of link—an ADHDer's life experience of coping with ADHD can consciously enter into the calculations here! Of course, this is not always possible, but if it succeeds, it helps you to perform nimbly where otherwise you would have to toil laboriously.

Be careful: the spontaneous linking in which positive hyperfocus is used to focus on an unloved task, can also have a destructive component. As a medical student, I was not yet aware of my ADHD. I couldn't care less about one particular subject—the lectures were boring. Unfortunately, attending the lectures was essential, because in the exams the lecturer asked exclusively about his own concepts that deviated slightly from the general scientific consensus.

I therefore used to sit in the venerable lecture hall with great distain. I could only concentrate on the stale explanations, because I was waiting for every tiny mistake the professor made, in order to confront him with it immediately. This hyperfocussed "game" went so far that when he refused to accept one of my objections, I asked him to think about it at home. The next day he admitted that I was right publicly, during the lecture. Looking back, I have the greatest respect for this professor, the magnanimity with which he took my justified but totally disrespectful criticism seriously and did not just throw me out. I probably wouldn't have been able to do that if I had been in his position.

Smart ADHDers, in whom thinking and associating in particular is unchecked, can expect additional deterioration in their performance. Even for subjects they are very interested in. When the school material offers **too little challenge**, their thoughts continue and the tasks to be completed tend not to get done. Occasionally, unusual solutions can be found for such situations (see Case Study 16).

Case Study 16
The School Pupil Who Could Only Do Mathematical Sums Listening to Music
Nalu was the daughter of Tom, a technician whom I was treating for his ADHD. Nalu was undoubtedly intelligent and lively. Mathematical and scientific questions in particular aroused her interest. Two years before completing school, she changed school. Suddenly, Nalu's marks in mathematics were now poor. Really bad.

Tom took a look at her exam papers with her. Astonished, he saw that Nalu had regularly solved only one task. The first one in each case, and this one completely correctly. She had left out the others, which were almost identical. Her explanation was:

Look, in the previous school, there were always different problems in an exam. That was no problem. But here, I'm supposed to prove the same thing five times, having already done this in the first task—I can't do it. That's when my thoughts drift away.

Nalu and her father Tom came up with a solution. They contacted the teacher and suggested that Nalu be allowed to listen to music with headphones during the exams. The teacher replied in horror that her grades were already at rock bottom, without music.

Patiently, Tom explained to the teacher how Nalu's ADHD works. That due to the boredom with the low mathematical challenge, Nalu's thoughts would drift far away, and as a result, it was almost impossible for her to concentrate. Music would occupy the brain of Nalu just enough to ensure that her thoughts would no longer stray too far (see also Sect. 4.2.1 as well as under Sect. 4.2.6: Case Study 4).

The teacher was persuaded to give it a try. And indeed, Nalu achieved top grades in mathematics again when listening to music.

The teacher's reaction was really good. Sensibly, he drew another conclusion from the story: he generally started to make the exams less monotonous, and for Nalu he always asked a tricky additional question.

Creating a good human environment is the best way to help everyone achieve their potential. When they start school, all children are still heavily dependent on having a supportive environment. With increasing maturity, this need is reduced.

In ADHDers, however, it has been shown that the dependence on good—or at least clear and non-negative—**human relationships** to teachers and trainers is stronger and also lasts longer. ADHDers should always remember this during their school career and vocational training.

For example, it has been shown that an ADHDer performs quite well in a school subject that is rather uninteresting for him, if the relationship with the teacher is good. If the teacher changes, and is followed by someone with whom there is no contact, the ADHDer's concentration and performance drop significantly.

Of course, this does not mean that the school or training position should be changed if the ADHDer performs poorly. But it is good to take these special circumstances into consideration. Of course, the same applies to all other relationships, friends, class group, other groups such as clubs and Internet communities, neighbourhoods and family.

ADHD can have **overlaps** with afflictions such as legasthenia, dyslexia, dyscalculia, or with autism spectrum disorders (Philipsen 2013). The conditions can be confused with each other. It is therefore always worthwhile finding out about the exact diagnosis, whether you are affected yourself, or as a parent.

Encore

In this context, I would also advise contacting reputable **self-help organisations** both for adult ADHDers, but especially for parents of adolescents with ADHD, or with the other above-mentioned afflictions. Particularly on the topic of vocational training and career choice.

The corresponding self-help organisations have extensive practical knowledge, which is sometimes neglected by medical and psychological specialists. You will also find that they have experience of dealing with school authorities, vocational trainers and know about the legal possibilities. And last but not least, mutual support is of central importance in a group of people who have had similar, difficult experiences.

9.2   Career Choice

For everyone, career choice is a decision that determines a great deal, if not everything, for your further path in life. With the term "decision", it is already clear that ADHDers easily have difficulties in this regard. In the abundance of information about all the exciting job profiles as well as the numerous branches in their thought trees, it is easy for ADHDers to get lost and it becomes difficult to decide. They can soon feel overwhelmed. Once more, the following applies: it's not that ADHDers think too little—they just think too widely.

The exception is those ADHDers who are lucky enough to have developed a special occupational interest at an early age, for whom no decision is therefore required anymore.

9.2.1   Take a Gap Year to Mature, if Necessary

If a delay in emotional-social development is apparent, a gap year may be useful after completing school education. Sometimes, even when the career choice is already clear. Certain professions require you to confront difficult situations, experiences and destinies. In some cases, a young person is not yet sufficiently mature in their personal development to cope with this.

Possible options include: an extra year in school; language stays, preferably in combination with a host family and/or a work assignment; various work placements; a year of voluntary or military service, if appropriate in your country of residence can be useful as a development step, as long as no war deployment is expected; volunteering in a social context; relief work to have genuine experience of the realities of life and much more.

The fear of losing a year is rarely justified. Looking at it from the perspective of your whole life, the time period of 1 year doesn't play a major role. In contrast, a well-planned gap year often offers a significant return on investment:

- Firstly, you are able to start vocational training or higher education study at a more mature age. This alone can help prevent early failure.
- Secondly, gap years give you a chance to expand your horizons and a wealth of experiences that you can draw upon for a lifetime.

9.2.2   Take Time and Develop a System to Aid Clarification

If we consider the two factors "delayed brain maturation" and "excessive amount of information to be processed", then it becomes clear that for ADHDers, choosing a career can require more effort (see above for the exception). It's therefore worth taking some time to do this.

Be careful: taking time is not the same as passively waiting.

On the other hand, it's important not to start any hectic overactivity. It's about giving yourself time to figure something out, to be able to perceive something, to let it "stew". This means that, despite the partially delayed development, it's nevertheless important to start thinking about career options at an early stage. This gives you time to play with, so to speak. However, one needs to be open to the process, and young people, owing to their age, often tend to pour scorn on the suggestions of adults. ADHD adolescents even more so.

Naturally, it's important to evaluate spontaneously expressed career wishes first. With these, it's important to find out why the young person finds them fascinating. Even more than with non-ADHDers, it is important to address these considerations without illusions. Today's online occupational information centres are a good place to start.

If the fascination of a profession and the facts about it match sufficiently, then the next step is to balance these with the young person's own requirements. Here too, it's important not to be under any illusions here:

- What can I do well or very well if necessary?
- In what areas am I not so talented?

- What do I enjoy doing?
- What do I not enjoy doing?
- Which of the things I don't enjoy doing, could I still do?
- To what extent?
- What are my personal no-goes?

- What kind of prestige is important to me in my profession?
- What are my ambitions in terms of earning opportunities?

The last two questions in particular are sometimes overlooked because they are considered ethically inferior, both by adolescents themselves and by adults. However, ignoring them would mean ignoring an existential reality in human life.

On this basis, the occupational fields in question can be narrowed down in a first step. Offering a system in this way makes a great deal of sense and acts as a kind of compass in today's huge range of job profiles.

9.2.3 Trial Working (Taster Day) Is Doubly Important: Tangible Rather Than Theoretical

Once the first considerations have been completed as described in Sect. 9.2.2, it is a matter of testing them tangibly in practical life.

TANGIBLE and PRACTICAL.

I cannot emphasise these two terms enough. As an ADHDer's imagination allows all kinds of possible and impossible scenarios, owing to the unchecked associations of the brain, it is doubly important to explore whether the reality corresponds sufficiently to the dreams.

On the one hand, checking these reveries serves to clarify whether a professional field is really as attractive as in the imagination of the ADHDer. Policework is not the same as a crime thriller, but involves a lot of routine tasks, waiting and writing numerous reports. Creating a constructive sense of disillusionment in the ADHDer is only one side of the story here.

The other side could be to discover that a desired occupation which you previously did not dared to consider, is *actually* suitable. Maybe your thinking is much better than you realised. Or perhaps you are more gifted in fine motoric skills than the required fine motoric training you received at kindergarten may have suggested.

In principle ADHDers can find their way more quickly in specific and practical situations than with theoretical considerations. There are unlimited possibilities for unchecked thinking in theory. On the other hand, the specific practical situation already provides a framework that helps to bring things into focus.

During these kinds of internships and taster days, you need to differentiate between the experiences linked to the *job itself*, and those more linked to the *people* you met when you were there. It is important to consciously distinguish between these two levels, so that your career choice is not accidental.

9.2.4   Own Choice or in the Slipstream of a Friend?

Sometimes the career choice encounters a stumbling block which, at first glance, is hardly noticeable: a young ADHDer chooses the same apprenticeship as their best friend or older sibling. Of course, this is not necessarily wrong, provided that the ADHDer actually wants to train for this career.

However, something else often lies behind it, especially if a firm career aspiration has not yet emerged. Good friendships and good sibling relationships are often even more meaningful for ADHDers than for non-ADHDers. Accordingly, the ADHDer may develop a subliminal fear of not being able to find their way in a new place without a familiar face. It's understandable if the career choice is therefore made in the shadow of a familiar person. This kind of coping mechanism has its price, because the career choice made in this way rarely fits. As a result, disappointment, demotivation and failure are unfortunately frequent.

> **Encore**
> Aligning yourself with a familiar person is quite reasonable in certain circumstances. As long as the trust is not blind. As long it is not abused to avoid taking responsibility for oneself. And, especially, as long as this coping mechanism is not exploited by the *people around you*.
>
> It is well known that young people are generally at risk of being seduced by allegedly overly large values. ADHDers with the above coping mechanism are particularly vulnerable in this regard. In addition to the usual adolescent

uncertainty and search for meaning, there is also an uncertainty that arises from the delayed development as well as from the unfiltered flood of data.

As a result, it is especially important for young ADHDers to be wary of all kinds of "saviours": fundamentalist-religious groups, whatever the religion; radical political groups, no matter which political persuasion; other ideologically extreme communities, no matter the direction; medical, psychological and esoteric communities with a guru cult and so on.

9.2.5 How Much Should I Say When Applying for an Apprenticeship/Trainee Position?

There is no universally valid answer to this question. I recommend that you think about this issue in a quiet moment, and weigh up the pros and cons in a pragmatic way. And above all, do not rashly communicate your ADHD (see Sect. 4.1). Because once you have published the information, you cannot take it back.

9.2.5.1 Disclosing at an Early Stage

For example, if the ADHD tends to be quite noticeable, if misunderstandings quickly arise in communication, if concentration and reliability regarding time are insecure, certain learning steps are slow and if the emotional-social deficit is pronounced, then concealing the ADHD would be grossly negligent. It is almost predestined that the young person will break off the apprenticeship early.

In these and comparable situations, it is necessary to inform superiors at an early stage. The young person should not only speak about the possible difficulties but communicate their wish—as long as it exists—to develop in these areas as fully as possible.

The support measures that the young person is receiving should be explained, whether it is psychotherapeutic support, coaching, drug treatment or other elements.

Similarly, the young person should explain the basic functionalities of ADHD to their superiors, such as the different learning curve. It is very important to point out the type of communication that is useful for an ADHDer. In particular how a supervisor can avoid triggering negative hyperfocus (see Sect. 6.1).

If the superior knows and respects these ADHD characteristics, he/she can still teach and criticise the apprentice *without any limitations*. As long as the apprentice can perceive the human acceptance of the supervisor, hefty criticism is also accepted. To put it briefly "hard but warm", or perhaps, the other way around is better, "if warmth exists, hardness can be easily accepted".

An open conversation also offers opportunities for the future training company: On the one hand to signal goodwill to the apprentice; on the other hand, to set out the limits of what is feasible. This is essential for *mutual* understanding.

Both contractual parties should receive something, but both must also offer something in return. This self-evident fact is sometimes forgotten by one party or the other.

It must be made clear to the apprentice that he has to achieve a certain level of performance. It is true that using the so-called "compensation of disadvantage" regulation, certain ADHD-related difficulties can be cushioned (see Sect. 9.3.3). For example, through a longer induction phase or additional time in exams. However, if the young person wants to complete the apprenticeship course, he must ultimately know and be able to do the same as the other candidates.

Of course, there are young people who have developed a very pronounced problem and who need more comprehensive support during their vocational training. In these cases, cooperation with state and private disability organisations becomes necessary. Fortunately, the government agencies are beginning to realise that the funds deployed in these areas are excellent, sustainable investments, both in human and in financial terms (Biedermann 2004). However, there is still very much to be done here.

9.2.5.2 Disclosing at a Late Stage or Not at All

The situation is different for ADHDers who are coping well with their ADHD. Especially in those who are less impulsive, are less distracted thanks to a high interest in their work, do not easily fall into negative hyperfocus and have already been able to learn to deal with their ADHD constructively. In such circumstances, disclosure is not necessary.

Of course, it is your own judgement and decision, if you decide to reveal your ADHD anyway. Especially in training companies with a positive, quasi-family atmosphere. If I generally advise a restrained tendency here, it is not because I want to foster an atmosphere of suspicious secrecy, nor do I want to trick the training company. It's just that information about one's own state of health, and especially about one's genetics, is subject to legally protected privacy. It should only be released after careful consideration. It can no longer be taken back.

However, if problems relating to ADHD do arise during the course of the apprenticeship, then I advise that you do not wait too long. Then a proactive approach would be advisable, in combination with the self-evident, but by no means defensive hint to your employer that at the beginning of the apprenticeship, you had no difficulties, which was why there was no reason to disclose the information.

9.2.6   Are There Legal Limitations Regarding ADHD in Particular Professions?

In Chap. 7, I explained about possible medications and their importance for professional life. I pointed out that country-specific career restrictions may exist with regard to so-called stimulants (e.g. methylphenidate, dexmethylphenidate, dexamphetamine, lisdexamphetamine, modafinil).

The presence of ADHD is not a fundamental obstacle to any profession. There is also no obligation to report to the employer. If in doubt, it is advisable to obtain specific information before starting an apprenticeship.

9.3   Education and Further Training

9.3.1   Summarised Overview of Apprenticeships and Higher Education Studies

I have summarised some considerations on vocational training and higher education study under the aspect of ADHD below. The list is not exhaustive, it only serves as rough orientation to be considered (Table 9.1).

Table 9.1 Compare apprenticeship and higher education study

	Apprenticeship	Higher education study
Advantages	– Specific tasks facilitate concentration and motivation – After a short time, satisfaction from experience of own work – Practical and theoretical learning go hand in hand – Working structures are largely predetermined and facilitate orientation	– Gives a certain freedom, curious and yet without responsibility, to explore the world and life – Allows prolonged adolescence to compensate for the ADHD-related delay in brain development
Disadvantages	– Too narrowly defined work structures can also trigger pubertal defiance – For some people, the move to a primary adult environment is too early owning to delayed development – This can (does not have to) lead to difficulties in adjusting	– Less strict structures of higher education study make orientation and work organisation more difficult – The loss of family structure when leaving the parental home can make self-organisation and self-structuring problematic – Possible difficulties in settling in a different city – The new local and student environment can distract from studies, as it is especially exciting
Compensation for disadvantage	– Possible	– Possible
To consider	– Entry into the world of work from the age of 15–16 – Delayed brain maturation continues to play a major role, there is still a certain emotional-social immaturity – The sometimes still childish attitude initially requires partially "parental" guidance by teachers, not just the "boss" model – Consider whether outing your ADHD is necessary and constructive or counterproductive	– Begins only from age 18 or later, brain somewhat more mature, but still emotionally socially more immature than those of same age – Risk of initially missing the connection to learning material due to the illusion that there is still endless time to learn – Conversely, there is also a risk of not integrating socially because of an excessive focus on studying

Fortunately today, the barriers between the different educational paths are permeable.

This is helpful to the way ADHD functions. Sometimes it is only when an ADHDer catches up in their developmental delay that the necessary seriousness in professional matters develops and therefore also the corresponding decisiveness (see Case Study 9).

Thus, after completing an apprenticeship via a vocational school-leaving certificate, it's possible to study later at a university of applied sciences. With additional examinations, one can also attend university teaching institutions. In addition, it is possible to achieve a formally recognised training status or a degree later in professional life with appropriate professional experience through in-service continuing education programmes such as CAS (Certificate of Advanced Studies), DAS (Diploma of Advanced Studies) and MAS (Master of Advanced Studies).

9.3.2 Learning and Swotting for Exams with ADHD

Learning takes a lot of effort, and this also applies to non-ADHDers. It is known as work. Learning has absolutely nothing to do with the film images of romantic mahogany libraries, green shining lampshades and heroically worked through nights, at the end of which a scientific breakthrough and the love of your life are always waiting.

Let's be honest: swotting for an exam can be boring, even if the opportunity to learn is a privilege. Of course, the acquisition of knowledge and the development of understanding are also uplifting. However, with a significant delay.

This delayed reward may be a bigger problem for ADHDers than for non-ADHDers. Without a direct stimulus in the moment—whether it's a direct interest in the moment or an immediate reward for your effort—it can be difficult to concentrate. However, other factors must also be taken into account for ADHDers with regard to learning and examinations (Rietzler and Grolimund 2018).

9.3.2.1 The Brutal Truth Is: Learning to Understand Is Not the Same as Learning for Exams

First it is necessary to face the obvious difference between the two forms of learning. This difference is not perceived by many ADHDers, let alone accepted (see Sect. 4.2.3 about apparent naivety).

- The first form is fundamental learning. Getting used to a topic, immersing yourself in it because you want to understand it. Wrestling for knowledge, turning the material over in your mind during discussions with other students and with the teachers. Defending the material—or tearing it apart—in a speech or a counterargument. Practising how to apply it, trying it out.

  This is learning for the sake of learning, in order to achieve knowledge and understanding, to grasp the essence of a topic and to be able to classify it to some extent in an overall understanding of the world and human life, in its causal contexts and the mutual impact on other fields. Gottfried Schatz (1936–2015), one of the most outstanding biochemists and thinkers, has wonderfully described this way of learning, researching and working in a column entitled "My secret university" (Schatz 2003).

- The second form is much more banal: swotting for exams. Nevertheless, it is an indispensable fact of life. The aim is to memorise given knowledge by heart and to reproduce it in the exams—mainly without having to think about it. Even at universities, numerous exams are now held only in multiple-choice procedures.

  This form of learning is all about passing an exam. And nothing else.

Many ADHDers, especially those who are very intelligent, do not perceive this difference or refuse to recognise it. For them, only the fundamental form of learning allegedly exists. This can sometimes have devastating consequences.

Encore

I can fully appreciate why people do not want to admit this difference. I was and am repeatedly tempted to ignore it myself and to consider only fundamental learning as acceptable. However, that would be wrong. Even memorised knowledge obviously has its uses.

On top of that, it is a banal fact that a developed society with a highly differentiated division of labour needs a way to be able to check knowledge and issue licences to practise certain occupations. On the other hand, one can and should of course discuss whether the selection of the knowledge to be tested and the examination methods are appropriate.

Of course, it is possible to pass an exam with fundamental learning, in other words, with the type of learning first described. Per se. However, there is usually not enough time to process all subjects comprehensively. How easy it is to immerse yourself in a subject, with the risk of getting lost in it, while neglecting other subjects.

Unfortunately, I have met numerous apprentices and students to whom exactly this has happened. At best, they lost a year or two in their training; at worst, they ended up with a feeling of resignation and complete rejection of this world.

Ultimately, it's about finding a balance—as so often in life—between the first fundamental and the second exam-oriented form of learning.

Striving for a balance does not mean that you are surrendering to sometimes trivial examination requirements. Rather, it allows both: reserving time for interesting, fundamental learning in selected topics as well as to complete sufficient exam learning. The main thing that results from this balance is the chance to pass exams, complete your training and acquire the licence to work in your chosen occupational field.

9.3.2.2 Realistic Learn Planning

The basic principle of learn planning is:

- The academic year or semester starts on the first day → so learning also starts on the first day.
- This means that individual parts of the learn planning are advantageously already determined beforehand. Namely, those that are doable in advance—with little effort. For example, setting up a system for organising documents, notes, scripts and books; or planning how to process new material weekly, from the very beginning, in manageable and predetermined portions. You can use the same method that I described in section "Using a Routine to Stop Thinking".
- In any case, it's a good idea to define for yourself pragmatically the balance between fundamental learning and swotting for exams at this early stage.
- The basic principle of learn planning also includes defining learning-free times, to allow your brain to recover—and this is indispensable. Time for leisure, for relationships, but also for tasks such as housework, organising or similar. Defined time windows give you an overview and mean that you are calmer.

Without a basic plan, you will be behind in a very short time, that is, within one to a few weeks. It is theoretically possible to catch up from this point. However, ADHDers feel this backlog according to the 1-2-3-too-much principle, the Mount Everest Syndrome (see Sect. 7.2), and it soon seems to be insurmountable. This demotivates them, leading to procrastination. They neglect both the fundamental learning and the swotting for exams (Grolimund 2018). They get a bad conscience which consumes energy, and in the end they panic and end up doing last-minute cramming for the exam.

Even if they pass the exam in this way, it doesn't bring much satisfaction as they still have considerable uncertainty in their specialist topics. Below I describe some tried-and-trusted methods on how to remain focussed on the material, avoid procrastination and stay "on the ball".

9.3.2.3 Learning Curve

If ADHDers want to learn something, it's a good idea for them to visualise the special ADHD learning curve. I described this in detail in Sect. 5.1.

As a reminder: being aware of this special type of knowledge acquisition can help you accelerate your own learning curve. The ADHD condition definitely does not mean an inability to prioritise and to filter, but merely that less automatic pre-filtering takes place. If you are aware of this, specific attention can be paid to getting an overview of the situation and focussing on a particular learning topic.

In this case, there's a chance you will be able to have your cake and eat it. This is one of the advantages of ADHD—if you know how to use it. More on this below, when it comes to different types of structure (Fig. 9.2).

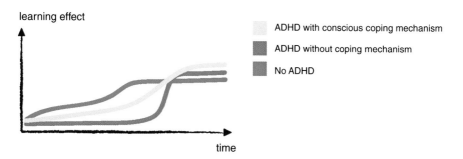

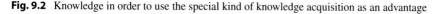

Fig. 9.2 Knowledge in order to use the special kind of knowledge acquisition as an advantage

> **Encore**
> The Swiss expression for the elegant English saying, "you can't have your cake and eat it" is "you can't keep your five francs and get the bread roll as well" or "man kann nicht den Fünfer und das Weggli haben".

9.3.2.4 Table of Contents as a Structure

- It sounds banal, but is often forgotten. The first thing you need is an overview of a topic that you need to learn.
- At the same time, we know that getting an overview is the central basic issue for every ADHDer.

Imagine that you are doing an apprenticeship as a cabinetmaker, and you need to familiarise yourself with the different types of wood. Full of interest, you open a textbook, read in fascination about Phoenician juniper timber, then about the bitternut tree, the incense-cedar, the European beech, the Nippon maple and the spruce. Probably not much of the information stays in your brain. And you haven't even got as far as important types of timber such as fir, oak and ash.

The first thing you need to do is get an initial overview. You need to classify the different types of timber, e.g. solid timber, chipboard, plywood, etc. In the individual types, there is another subdivision, e.g. solid timber in coniferous trees and deciduous trees.

As the title of this subchapter has already revealed, the table of contents for a textbook can be used to get an initial overview—it shows the division of a topic into the relevant areas.

- It's a good idea to make a paper copy of the table of contents and highlight the relevant chapters in one colour and the subchapters in a second colour. You could shade chapters and subchapters that are interesting but insignificant in grey to indicate that they can be ignored.

In this way, an entire field of expertise shrinks to a clear, manageable size, with a recognisable structure.

- Subsequently, the rough structure of the specialist topic created by the chapters sinks into your brain. As soon as you want to start studying one of the chapters, let the structure of the subchapters also sinks in to your brain.
- Place this printed table of contents, reworked with colours, in a clearly visible place next to the book or, in the case of e-books, next to the computer, where it offers you—constantly in the corner of your eye—a focus point for classifying what you have just read.

If you approach learning in this way, the details you read do not hang incoherently in the air, but are absorbed *and* stored in context from the very beginning. Do you remember? ADHDers find it easier to remember facts if they exist in a plausible context, not just isolated data sets, and form stories to a certain extent.

9.3.2.5 Personal Experiences and Specific Examples as Orientation Structure

Experiences you have had yourself stick better than pure theory. This is a well-known fact when it comes to learning.

Your own experiences also serve as anchor points where you can park theoretical knowledge. Or as lighthouses that offer an orientation structure in the ocean of knowledge. No matter which image you choose, it helps to internalise the dry theory using memorable experiences.

In vocational training, practical experience is a fundamental part of the training system. This is less true for higher education study. It may be worthwhile completing additional work placements in your relevant field of study, or taking on a small auxiliary job alongside your studies related to your specialist subject. This auxiliary structure will help to anchor the theory better in your brain.

Anecdotes, cartoons, jokes and classic memory aids such as "Never Eat Shredded Wheat" to remember the sequence of points on a compass (North, East, South, West) can also work in a similar way to tangible experiences. They all form emotional engrams which make very robust orientation points.

Some of the strongest emotional engrams that help us to learn are mistakes we make ourselves. Of course, they do not have to be brought about intentionally—they will happen anyway to a more than sufficient degree. But then they can offer a lasting learning effect. In this respect, it's important to take the observation attributed to Jean-Paul Sartre (1905–1980) to heart, "One should commit no stupidity twice, the variety of choice is, in the end, large enough".

9.3.2.6 Group Learning as Structure

Another structure that can be particularly important for ADHDers is linking up with a study group. Of course, one naturally needs to be part of the group first. So, it's important to start making contacts here early in every year of training.

Encore

ADHDers may take longer to find their way around in a new environment such as an apprenticeship or a degree course at university, so they can easily miss hooking up with a study group.

But knowing about this will help you to consciously counteract it. To do this, keep the following banal points in mind:

- The longer you have not approached anyone in a new environment, the more difficult it will be.
- And the chances of finding suitable colleagues at a later date become smaller.
- If you also know that your non-ADHD colleagues are also insecure at the beginning, then this point of reference will help you to proactively approach others on the first day of your vocational college or university semester.

Be smart, and take advantage of the small window of time in which practically *everybody* feels insecure! ADHDers, who have a clear orientation about the situation can often make a surprising number of good contacts. Even those who regard themselves as shy.

There are many advantages of a study group. These can be decisive for ADHDers:

- By working together in a group, the tendency to invest excessively in a single subject and get lost in it is reduced. It is much more likely that you will stick to the collegially agreed learning plan.
- In the same way, you are less likely to fluctuate between excessive last-minute swotting followed by a passive collapse. Your continuity in learning is better.
- If you don't know something, you can ask a direct question. You save yourself from having to do tedious, boring and demotivating research on your own. Procrastination and wasting time are unnecessary.
- And vice-versa: if you explain a fact to a group member, your own knowledge is solidified because you have to be clear about it in your own mind. What's more, it's only by explaining that you discover previously unrecognised gaps—and are then able to fill them.
- Regular contact and discussions in the group give you continuous orientation about your own learning progress in comparison with your colleagues. This classification is decisive in helping you to feel secure, to continue learning more or less calmly, even to take breaks in order to recover and to be able to face the exams reasonably calmly.

9.3.2.7 Technical Aids

From a technical point of view, ADHDers have an abundance of aids at their disposal these days. Sometimes this abundance is actually problematic: it can seem impossible to figure out which are the right apps to use.

As an ADHDer, always remember the principle that the goal is not to find the perfect and ideal tool, but one that is sufficient. And one that is easy to use. Often, therefore, it is simply a good idea to use something that a colleague is already using, both in terms of hardware and software.

Currently, a powerful tablet that functions like a laptop with a keyboard and that also allows pen input seems to me to be ideal for use in vocational training.

Spend enough time determining which apps and programmes you want to use. For example, it is important to be able to share content with colleagues and work together on a project.

I recommend a tried and tested notebook programme such as Evernote or OneNote as a basis. In it, notes, scripts, photos, sketches and more can be stored in an orderly fashion—and, above all, found again. Ideally you should be able to annotate texts with the pen so that you can really work as if using a notebook. Project work can be structured, planned and managed. Depending on the situation, special programmes for project management such as Trello, ClickUp, Zenkit or others may be helpful.

Digital possibilities are developing rapidly. In addition to the notebook programmes that are currently considered a basic tool, special applications can be found for practically everything. For example, to-do apps, apps to structure your learning workload, flashcard apps, mind map apps and other learning apps.

Podcasts of lectures that can be conveniently listened to on your mobile phone when travelling are becoming increasingly popular. YouTube videos, online lectures, online study groups and much more can be used.

BUT be careful:

As we all know, it's very easy to get lost in the digital world extremely quickly. Just select a few programmes that you can then learn and work with. In the same sense, don't look at a thousand lectures on a subject, but just at those from your teaching institution.

Encore

If you do prefer to write by hand, collect notes in binders and want to lug around several books, then of course you are welcome to do so.

Nevertheless, check whether this is really what you want, or whether you are secretly afraid that you won't be able to cope with the technology. If the latter applies, I suggest you familiarise yourself with the technology and if necessary, even attend a course. Give a friend the chance to help you out here. It's definitely worth it.

9.3.3 Possibilities, Boundaries and Pitfalls of a Compensation for Disadvantage Status

9.3.3.1 Fundamental Comments on Compensation for Disadvantage Status

With ADHD, you have—to some extent and in some countries—a legal right to so-called "compensation for disadvantage". This means a partial compensation of the disadvantage that may be present owing to your ADHD (compared to non-ADHDers) during your vocational training and in university exams.

This compensation for disadvantage is based on country-specific disability equality laws. According to the law, ADHD is considered a disability. As a general statement about ADHD, this is extremely questionable. However, it is correct with regard to the conditions of vocational training and examinations, which are aimed at non-ADHDers.

Compensation for disadvantage can only be granted where there is a disadvantage owing to the diagnosed disability, but the required cognitive and subject-related requirements for the career in question are also present *simultaneously*. Deciding where the boundaries lie here is not always easy.

Compensation for disadvantage does not mean that an ADHDer needs to know less and be able to do less at the end of the vocational training. A misunderstanding here would represent a devastating pitfall of compensation for disadvantage.

A diagnosis of ADHD does not automatically lead to measures of compensation for disadvantage. This wouldn't make sense. It would suggest that those ADHDers who are not disadvantaged by the "configuration" of their ADHD in education also have limitations. This suggestion would be a hindrance rather than a help.

Compensation for disadvantage must therefore be applied for and justified on an individual basis. This regulation may sometimes be annoying because it requires a degree of effort. But rights also entail responsibilities.

In this sense, the ADHD compensation for disadvantage during vocational training refers to the following key points:

- There is a developmental delay, especially in emotional and social areas. It is advisable for the ADHDer to be accommodated to an appropriate extent and, if necessary, to have additional support (mentoring). It will no longer play a significant role in later professional life, when the ADHDer catches up on their developmental delay (see Sect. 9.1.1).
- The fact that pre-filtering of information and thoughts takes place less automatically means that the ADHDer requires more time to get an overview. This has a particularly strong effect in a vocational training situation where completely new learning content has to be classified every day (see Sect. 5.1). It therefore makes sense to make more time available to absorb learning content. In later professional life, this will hardly play a role any more, because you can classify new situations on well-known professional terrain. ADHDers often achieve this even faster at a later date than non-ADHDers.

- Less pre-filtering of information and thoughts, as described above, means that you need more time in examination situations, which should be compensated for. In addition, unchecked thinking occasionally leads to ADHDers discovering the smallest ambiguities in questions, and then thinking about them far too much. As well as a loss of time, this can also lead to ADHD-related misunderstanding. To a certain extent, having the opportunity to make a simple request to clarify the task is appropriate here.
- Increased distractibility and difficulties in concentrating are a hindrance under teaching and examination conditions. The nature of the distraction in the classroom and in exams in no way corresponds to the working situations in the profession. It therefore makes sense to take these circumstances into account during the vocational training and examinations.

The justifications that must be included in the applications for compensation for disadvantage ensure that neither the trainers nor the trainees have the misconception that ADHDers are gaining preferential treatment here.

The regulatory requirements for submitting applications for compensation for disadvantage are extremely diverse. At some educational institutions, a simple medical certificate submitted just before the exam is sufficient. For other institutions, a broad-based application must be submitted before the beginning of the semester which ends with the examination in question. It is definitely important to find out about the applicable regulations at an early stage.

9.3.3.2 Compensation for Disadvantage Status for Everyday Situations During Apprenticeship and Higher Education Study

During everyday working situations in **vocational training**, it is possible to compensate ADHD-related difficulties on an individual basis. For example:

- Allowing more time for a certain task to be carried out independently.
- Increased possibility of consulting at the beginning of a rotation with another department; mentoring that extends beyond the scope usually offered.
- Help in getting an overview of the tasks to be completed in 1 day; more support in organising tasks.
- Spending more time going over the working day or the working week afterwards.
- And other measures, depending on the individual situation.

The measures should be included in an overall plan. Here, structure should be given from external parties only where necessary. The goal is for the ADHDers to take over most of the structuring themselves over time. If necessary, e.g. when changing to a new department, the support will be ramped up again at short notice.

In the case of **higher education study**, other forms of compensation for disadvantage can be effective. For example:

- Stronger support from the student counselling service in organising your studies.
- Reserving a place at the front of the lecture hall in order to be less distracted by fellow students.

- Increased professional mentoring, either across the board or only in certain subjects.
- And other measures, depending on the individual situation.

Sometimes it's not possible to discern which measures are necessary at first glance. Seen from another person's point of view, they may seem to concern insignificant areas. Areas that may seem implausible to non-ADHDers.

For example, a highly motivated student showed pronounced difficulties in concentrating during a heavily attended, centrally important lecture series in the venerable, tightly packed lecture hall of her university. It was only after some time that it became clear that she had an unfiltered, enhanced sense of smell (see Controlling and dosing, Sect. 3.2.2). Squeezed into the old lecture hall, it was hard for her to avoid the whiffs of various "odours". She received permission to reserve the places next to her for "odourless" fellow students (i.e. not the onion or garlic consumers; nor the ones "allergic" to taking a shower; nor the over-enthusiastic perfumers).

9.3.3.3 Exam-Related Compensation for Disadvantage Status
Compensation for disadvantage for exams usually concerns two areas:

- The possibility of taking the exam in a separate room to reduce ADHD-related increased distraction.
- Extended time frame, up to 25%, to cover the ADHD-related increased time requirement described above.

Other measures may also be useful and can be requested with justification. For example, in handwritten exams (yes, they still exist) the right to write on the computer if fine motoric difficulties lead to illegible writing. Or the opportunity for simple clarification questions on how to understand a task.

9.3.4   ADHD-Basics for Surviving the Day of Your Exam and Passing It

It's well worth getting an overview of how to approach exams with ADHD. The importance of such a plan is illustrated by the following case study:

Case Study 17
The Student Who Trained His ADHD in Particular, After Messing Up an Exam—And Won
Many years ago, Mike, a very bright business student, came to me for treatment. Somehow, he had managed to cope with his ADHD. He knew he was intelligent. His achievements at academic high school had been outstanding. Actually, he only came because he had to switch to an adult psychiatrist for the sake of his age to carry on receiving prescriptions of methylphenidate.

It seemed that he suffered from typical hidden, ADHD-related self-doubt, something which he himself found implausible. Meaning that he doubted himself even more. Mike skilfully hid his doubts by proving himself to be a master of humorous witty verbal debates.

One could almost have suspected narcissistic traits, but he did not show any of the typical narcissistic power games—only pure joy in having good contact with the person he was speaking to. He impressively described the warm, albeit sometimes exuberant situation in his birth family with deep and resilient relationships.

ADHD was diagnosed early in childhood. Mike received drug treatment. ADHD was hardly ever explained to him, not even later in adolescence. Without much discussion, he was prescribed analytically focussed psychotherapy for years.

This therapy was a strange prerequisite for the prescription of the methylphenidate, which had been imposed by his child psychiatrist. Analytical psychotherapy is not the treatment of choice for ADHD unless there is a significant unconscious problem at the same time. There was no evidence of this.

From childhood to adolescence, Mike uncomplainingly attended sessions that completely passed him by—which did nothing to increase his trust in psychotherapy. The therapist propagated a mother problem, probed for years—and found nothing. Mike resigned himself to having to put up with the sessions now and then. In typical ADHD fashion, he accepted the prerequisite set by the psychiatrist as a given.

When he came to me, Mike was convinced that he had to keep talking about his mother as a matter of course. I, on the other hand, suggested sessions to him where he could explore how his ADHD functioned but stressed that the talks were, of course, voluntary. Surprised by this casualness, Mike was relieved. For the time being, he only wanted infrequent progress discussions.

This did not change as his first university exams approached. He saw no need for ADHD-specific exam preparation, given his achievements at school.

The only thing is that the amount of material, the learning itself as well as the exams, is completely different at university than at school. Although he had mastered the material very well (he had simply learned "everything"), he totally flunked the assessment exams.

Mike remembered how I had offered him a chance to understand how his ADHD functions and apply the knowledge to exams. Extremely motivated, he now concentrated on this, asked questions, described his own observations and voraciously absorbed the specialist explanations.

It turned out that in the stress of the exams he had very quickly lost track of the tasks. Immediately, he doubted his learning success. When he didn't understand a task, he went into negative hyperfocus and panic, lost valuable time and made all kinds of careless mistakes in the rush.

Mike quickly realised that he didn't need to learn anything extra for his exam subjects. But he sought every opportunity to understand himself and the way his ADHD functioned better, and to regulate himself more reliably. Above all, he practised how, even in the midst of negative hyperfocus, he could recognise this and work his way out of it. He continued to take the ADHD medication in the same way as earlier.

At the second attempt, he passed the assessment exams with very good grades. In the meantime, Mike has completed his business studies with a master's degree, without ever having to repeat another exam. Moreover, he completed an extremely demanding supplementary education course and has established himself in the business world.

Below I sketch out a structure for exams that has proved to be helpful to many ADHDers. Of course, you can and should adapt it to your own situation (Table 9.2).

Table 9.2   Basics about the exam and exam day

Preparation phase (weeks/ months)	– Learning (see Sect. 9.3.2) – Submit if needed an application for compensation for disadvantage on time (see Sect. 9.3.3) – Do not miss registration for the exam; do it early so that you have decided, and do not waste any more energy thinking about this decision. – Prepare for the exam – Mental training on how to cope if you lose track of things during the exam (see sections "General Orientation in Situations" and "Overview of the Relevance of the Tasks to Be Completed") – Mental training on how to deal with negative hyperfocus, if you get into it during the exam (see Sect. 6.4) – Familiarise yourself with the route to the location of the exam **Evening before** – Plan the day of the exam (before, during *and* after the exam) – Get clothes, food, isotonic drink, any medicines, writing materials, papers and necessary documents ready
Day of the exam: Time before the exam	When you wake up on the day of the exam, immediately keep two basic focus points in mind: – **First**: I have learned the material and can "do it" *sufficiently* – **Second**: Keep in mind in how many hours the exam will be over. Visualising the end time point helps you to focus and stay on course – Fill the time before the exam with banal activities, however they should not be tiring – As far as possible, try to avoid having any long, empty waiting time immediately before the exam. Otherwise, the thought trees will spread out and there is a danger you will be thrown off track and panic – If you are being treated with stimulants, make sure that the level also covers the time leading up to the exam, as evenly as possible. Otherwise: sprawling thought trees, uncertainty and fear – Get close to the exam location at an appropriate early stage to prevent additional stress due to heavy traffic or delays in public transport

Exam	**Start**
	– When you receive the tasks, do not start immediately, but first get an overview
	– If possible, do an easy task first, thereby gaining initial certainty (see Sect. 7.2.1)
	Getting stuck and blackout
	– If a task does not seem solvable, create an inner distance to it briefly. Do not get too involved in this task, otherwise you will lose time and your uncertainty will increase. It is better to solve another task first
	– If you get stuck on a question that you know in principle but have just lost track of ("blackout"), proceed according to the mental training above:
	• If you lose track of things because you are **thinking too widely**: think for a moment, what kind of question do I "hear" internally when I slowly read the task word by word, almost without thinking?
	• If **negative hyperfocus**: free yourself from it. For details, see Sect. 6.4. If you do not succeed in doing this in a useful period of time, then skip the question and come back to it later
	– The time required for this is not lost; rather, it reduces anxiety and releases energy again
	Medication management
	– Medication management should ensure a steady level throughout the entire time of the examination
	– It's very important to prevent the medication level from falling below its level of effectiveness, otherwise rebound phenomena may cause a massive drop in performance
	– But equally important: Medication overdose must be prevented, otherwise hyper-nervousness or, if the overdose is even higher, drowsiness
	For examinations lasting several hours:
	– Drink something regularly (isotonic drinks, energy drinks, etc.). Lack of fluid reduces concentration
	– Make sure that your blood sugar level does not drop. Glucose, bananas, dried fruits, nuts, salty snacks, etc.
	– Take a 1–2-min break regularly (every 30–40 min); relax for a while; focus your thoughts on something completely different (such as the silence in the mountains or the roaring celebration of a goal in the stadium)
Day of the exam: Time after the exam	– In the seconds after handing in the exam; in other words, *before* the adrenaline drops, and the thought trees expand into infinity again: briefly assess whether you have done well. Hold this impression and let it sink into your memory
	– You should accept that, with increasing distance from the exam and through the conversations with colleagues, all possible and impossible uncertainties will arise. Take note of these as unpleasant and inevitable, otherwise focus on the first impression, if it is positive
	– If you had a "bad feeling" directly before or after handing in the exam, then immediately try to focus on the mantra "it can come out one way or another, I only know it when I know it", and distract yourself as soon as possible
	– In any case, carry out a previously planned activity. It's often good to meet up with friends, partner or family (as long as they are constructive people). Activities such as sports, an excursion, dancing, game evening, cooking or movie night; anything that prevents you from thinking that is unchecked or too far

9.3.5 Planning and Completing Written Work on Time

Mark Twain (1835–1910): *If it weren't for the last minute, nothing would get done.*

Mark Twain aptly characterises an experience that ADHDers know particularly well. Extensive written papers are a major hurdle for many of them.

Imaginative ideas with far-reaching associations and profound considerations, but no idea how and where the starting point should be set, limit the spectrum, on the one hand; empty ideas, on the other. Both are followed by a nervous passivity which leads to a rush of panic as the deadline approaches.

I do not intend to present a comprehensive guide on how to write papers/essays/theses here, but only to highlight some aspects that are particularly helpful for ADHDers.

Fundamentally, it's about gaining an overview and orientation—as always in ADHD. This concerns various areas.

9.3.5.1 Purpose of the Paper to Be Written

These kinds of written papers primarily exist for passing an exam. Proving your ability or knowledge is only of secondary importance.

From a pragmatic point of view, the quality of such work determines your further career path in only a few disciplines, for example, if you aspire to have a university career, or if, as an aspiring journalist, you succeed in creating an outstanding reportage as your final thesis.

I am not advocating specialist or academic sloppiness here. It's simply that I want to acknowledge that after completing vocational training, proving yourself on an everyday basis is the most important criterion for a successful career.

9.3.5.2 Type, Scope and Structure of the Paper to Be Written

Strange but not surprising for those who know a lot about ADHD: ADHDers assume en masse that every written paper, whether it is a specialisation in the third year of an apprenticeship or a dissertation, must reach at least the level of a Nobel Prize-winning habilitation thesis.

Encore

When working on a partial aspect of the first Kappel War in the sixteenth century (the Zurich Reformer Zwingli against the Catholics of Central Switzerland; the war was settled without a battle with a milk soup dinner), the context of all religious wars at that time should be worked out, at the very least, and from this, completely new perspectives on their significance for the development of the 30 Year War in the following century (several million dead) should be derived. Including information on its impact on the architecture and settlement structure of the villages in the Lower Engadine, with differences between Reformed and Catholic villages still visible today, which could allow a digression about the role of the Habsburgs…

If it is difficult to find the right dimension in the abundance of unfiltered, possible variants and ideas, the maximum is assumed to be the allegedly minimum reference value—in other words, one tends to overcompensate. It's better to not to do this.

In brief:

- Keep in mind the level that a paper needs to be. A bachelor's thesis is a bachelor's thesis, should be a bachelor's thesis and nothing else.
- Define the topic to be covered within these limits. As a rule, a small partial aspect of a topic should be dealt with properly. Discuss this with your supervisor, and please: do not tempt him to grant you a more extensive question.
- Take a look at the specifications of your training institution, both its scope and structure.

The scope is predetermined. For example: a bachelor's thesis is usually around 50 pages (without attachments), limited to a maximum of one hundred. Remember, the minimum must be achieved, not the maximum. Less is more—even the most interested professor appreciates finishing his work for the day in a timely manner.

The structure of written papers is also usually predetermined. For example: introduction, formulation of a question, theory, methodology, results, discussion, conclusions, directories.

- Write the appropriate headings in your word processing programme.
- Assign a corresponding proportion of the available (empty) pages to each chapter.

In no time, you can get a visual overview in this simple way.

You thereby realise, not only intellectually but also emotionally, that the task is doable, you do not have to think too far nor go back as far as Adam and Eve. The work no longer appears to be Mount Everest (see Sect. 7.2).

And with the overview, you can see that the small number of empty pages per chapter can be filled, even if you may be devoid of ideas. When you realise that the work is manageable, this even awakens your desire to get started.

9.3.5.3 Overview of Time Available

In addition to the content, it's always necessary to have an overview regarding time available to improve reduced work organisation capabilities (Sobanski and Alm 2004). It is worthwhile drawing a timeline at the very beginning, and roughly dividing up the tasks along it.

- **Immediately** you should complete the **overview**, in order to establish the purpose, nature, scope and structure of the work, as described above. This prevents the task from mutating into Mount Everest in your imagination.

Another **immediate task** is to create a **list** of the material, literature, documents, interview dates, laboratory or workshop times, etc. Place orders, reserve dates, reserve times.

- Define relatively small **intermediate** goals into manageable portions, in a fixed routine. Small portions of work allow you to start along the path more easily, rather than procrastinating. In sum, the intermediate goals achieved in small steps create a solid foundation for the paper to be written. This gives you motivation.
- Firmly define and schedule **non-working hours**. Be clear on when is it time to recuperate or do housework or other activities. This makes it easier to stay on the ball.
- **Reserve times** and **full-time commitment**: only plan reserve times from the middle of the entire period. Reserve times are necessary, there are always additional things to do or energy-free phases to compensate for. Realistically expect fluctuations between periods of energy boost and lethargy. In other words: no illusory planning! Also determine when the final phase begins with full-time commitment.

And here, too, the following applies: above all, the work must be finished and of sufficiently good quality. It only makes sense to strive for outstanding quality if the additional time and energy required are realistically available.

9.3.5.4 People as Important Aids for Orientation and Organisation

I have pointed out several times how important other people are for ADHDers, especially in Chaps. 5, 6 and 8. To summarise, they have helpful effects in the following areas:

- **Focus:** when discussing things with another person, you can quickly gain an overview in an overabundance of information and thoughts.
- **Self-worth:** being able to perceive one's own value more clearly in a constructive comparison to the other person and through requested feedback.
- **Organisation and implementation:** to be able to implement a plan better by being connected to someone.

All three areas play a role in the creation of a longer paper. The pièce de résistance is often the implementation of a plan. Different people play a role in this.

Firstly, it is important to select from any **mentors** available at an institution the ones who are most likely to offer support in the areas where difficulties exist.

If you have trouble narrowing down the field to a manageable dimension when choosing a topic, then a mentor who speaks unabashedly common sense is recommended. Someone who is not afraid to set limits for you—in other words, exactly what you have difficulties with. At the same time, the supervisor should ideally be a person you value, from whom you can accept boundary-setting and criticism.

Of course, it takes a huge portion of luck for such a mentor to be available. But here, too, the following applies: it is not about finding the ideal mentor, but the one who suits you sufficiently. After all, the success in writing the paper depends above all on you—fortunately!

Secondly, it is worth considering who and how someone from your **private environment** can be helpful. Here I do *not* mean that someone writes the paper for you.

Rather, it is about wondering who you can orientate yourself around. Who can help you with organisational tasks. After that, it is necessary to check whether the person of your choice is ready to take on this task. If so, the form of support must be discussed openly. If this step is ignored, misunderstandings easily arise, or the accompanying person gets the impression of being taken advantage of.

Often a little structural help is enough.

Case Study 18
The Eternal Student
Rolf was a classic eternal student. In times before the Bologna Reform, when many degree programmes were completed with a licentiate, he spent years working on his licentiate paper. He had already been teaching history at an academic high school for a long time. However, as he didn't have a degree, he only received the salary of a substitute teacher. This was a financial disaster.

He had collected and sorted vast amounts of material, he knew how to defend his thesis well, he had developed and refined exciting considerations and cross-connections. Everything had long been ready to be cast into written form.

His imagination was rigidly focussed on the fact that he had to be absolutely undisturbed and without distraction for this to succeed. After all, he had ADHD. So, he retreated to his apartment. No one was allowed to visit him, not even his girlfriend. The telephone and internet were mostly switched off.

It was just that as soon as he sat down at his desk, he inevitably got distracted. Nothing seemed to help.

The situation was reversed through a chance observation, when his girlfriend fell ill with stomach flu. She did not want to be alone and temporarily moved in with him. During the day, she usually slept, drank tea, ate rusks, otherwise she did nothing.

Rolf was initially annoyed that his allegedly necessary stimulus isolation had been disturbed. However, for the first time, his writing started to flow. Almost spontaneously he managed to bash out the formulations that had long been present in his head into the computer.

Soon Rolf realised that the presence of the girlfriend did not distract him, but helped him not to get lost in the ADHD-related infinity of possible thoughts. She helped him with the minimal "disturbance" to keep his orientation, to concentrate and to translate into writing what he had previously thought about (see Sect. 4.2.1).

As a result, he agreed with that his partner should stay in his apartment whenever possible. She was relieved in several ways. She was no longer kept at a distance, had the opportunity to do something for Rolf and was glad that the eternal student at her side was progressing with his licentiate.

The licentiate paper was finished in a few weeks.

Thirdly, you can consider targeted **structural and organisational help** from professionals. There is a wide range of **coaching** offers for bachelor, master or diploma theses. Some of these are serious, highly professional and accredited services.

However, there are also types of support which violate the rules for the preparation of theses, including illegal practices such as ghost-writing and plagiarism aids.

I absolutely do not recommend these kinds of services. Never forget: the affidavit, which is customary for theses, regarding compliance with the rules applicable at your training institution, is legally binding. If you violate it, your degree will be revoked and you may face possible further legal consequences.

9.4 Procrastination in Further Training, Career Planning and Other Occupational Projects

Despite all conceivable creativity and innovativeness, ADHDers are sometimes extremely persistent in procrastinating (Rist et al. 2011), in the preservation what is familiar to them. Why is this so?

- **Firstly**, this happens because of the central ADHD mechanism. If unweighted information and thoughts increase to a critical level, ADHDers can lose track of things and small tasks seem overpowering. Consequently, these are postponed or not even tackled (see Sect. 7.2).

- **Secondly**, areas are affected in which there is no direct personal interest. For example, I know ADHDers who work with completely outdated computer programmes. Not because they can't afford a new version, but simply because they have neither interest nor desire to deal with this situation.
- **Thirdly**, ADHDers tend to "freeze" in their everyday lives if an activity in itself does not affect the current moment. For example, organising a vacation, finally meeting a friend again, or finally doing something to find a partner.

They often never get around to these kinds of things. Not because they are not interested in them. But because *RIGHT NOW at this moment* something else has to be done. A task—at best, an everyday one—stands out so much at this moment that everything is focussed on it.

As soon as the everyday task is completed, the condition turns into dull languor which, in turn, *right now at this moment* also stands out, meaning that the ADHDer does not get around to doing what he actually wants to do (see the exhausting *Should I do it today or first tomorrow; why didn't I already do it yesterday* under Sect. 5.2.5).

This third type of procrastination plays a big role in working life in the medium- and long-term. Specialist advanced training, taking planned career steps or other professional projects are missed.

If countermeasures are not taken, the career path develops randomly, depending on what just happens to crop up. The constantly changing everyday requirements in professional and private life distract from fundamental and longer-term projects.

In addition, if typical ADHD self-doubt is also present, important steps of further training and development are missed, and suitable career opportunities are rejected.

This problem should be taken seriously as it causes great damage to many ADHDers. This unfolds not only financially, but also in all areas of professional and private life, as well as the satisfaction and identification with one's own career path.

It doesn't have to be like this. Precisely because of the serious consequences, you should clarify at an early stage whether action needs to be taken here (see also the following case study).

9.4.1 Living Appointment Calendar

Sometimes email and organisation programmes such as Outlook® are very helpful for managing appointments and tasks. They reliably remind you of tasks to be completed.

But: when it comes to important matters that are not urgent at that moment, many ADHDers deliberately ignore the alarms and reminders of these kinds of programmes.

Reminders and alarms work better when they come personally from a real flesh and blood person. A person whom you have already met face to face, whose eyes you have looked into. As with "Here's looking at you, kid" the legendary farewell spoken by Rick (Humphrey Bogart) to Ilsa (Ingrid Bergmann) in the classic film *Casablanca* (Wallis et al. 1942).

There is a greater connection. A kind of real live appointment calendar, one could almost speak of a "living" Outlook®.

This person-related principle can be used to advantage to prevent procrastination. It is especially useful for medium-term projects such as planning and completing further training, or other occupational projects.

Encore
It can be useful to implement the procedure described below in cooperation with a professional coach.

At an astonishingly low cost:

As a rule, two sessions are required to prepare the first project through a coach. Afterwards, usually only short phone calls of maximum 1–2 min are necessary. Further projects with the same coach require only one preparation session. So overall, a small amount of time, which remains financially within a manageable framework.

Detailed description of the specific procedure: in the desired case, the doctor or therapist will arrange a joint **first appointment** with the ADHDer and the coach in the practice. This appointment is to enable the parties to get to know each other, creating a mutually acknowledged basis and acceptance. Discussion should centre on the functioning of ADHD, the individual problems and the background to the chosen procedure.

In a **second appointment**, the ADHDer and the coach meet without the doctor or therapist. They define the individual areas of focus for the procedure. A concrete, detailed schedule is drawn up for an initial project. It is a classic task plan with deadlines for intermediate goals to be achieved.

The individual tasks that are to be remembered in this way must be defined completely pragmatically. These can be the most banal small tasks, such as "call Mr XY now and make an appointment", or also bigger assignments.

The decisive factor here is that you can identify those subtasks for which you need a personal reminder call. You do this by taking a pragmatic look at your own no-goes (see Sect. 7.3).

Shortly before something is to be done—in the following example the task is to pick up the phone, call the architect and confirm the proposed calendar weeks for your house renovation—the coach calls you.

This call is of extremely short duration. Its purpose—based on the binding nature of the mutual relationship—is to remind you of the execution of the task and give you the start impulse. Immediately afterwards, the task is completed without delay. Depending on the agreement, the coach will be notified that you have completed the task.

Encore

It is important that absolutely nothing is discussed in these phone calls. The only purpose of these telephone calls is to act as a personalised reminder and to trigger the start impulse. The "no-discussion rule" has proved to be essential. Otherwise, too often a conversation arises in which you tie yourself in knots, lose track of things, return to old misinterpretations of your alleged worthlessness, lose energy, become demotivated and end up postponing the task.

After a dry reminder call, on the other hand, the motivation, which is based on personal contact, is sufficient to complete the task immediately. Firstly, this increases your self-esteem, and secondly, it encourages you to tackle further hurdles without delaying them.

Depending on your needs, a reminder call can be arranged the evening before, so that the task for the next day is already fixed as immovable and of course in the back of your mind.

In this way, you are able to implement successfully even larger projects that have repeatedly fallen by the wayside, step by step.

It makes sense to start this kind of approach with only one project. More can be added, step by step; ideally your self-organisation technique can become a habit. Of course, you are also free to enter into this kind of cooperation in the long-term, to take out a subscription for a kind of "living appointment calendar" with a coach.

Case Study 19
The Brave Tailor

Florian was an elegantly, corpulent man in his late forties. Elegant because, as an ingenious tailor, he could skilfully make his male curves disappear under an elegant suit.

In addition to men's tailoring, he also worked as a ladies' couturier. With a flair for fleetingly implied extravagance, he designed stylish clothes for men and women. Even I, who am happy wearing jeans and a T-shirt, began to think about my wardrobe, but found Florian's prices a good excuse to keep things as they were.

Florian put his heart and soul into his creations and his desire for quality craftsmanship was absolute. It was important to him to offer his tailor-made garments in his own shop in the city centre. For reasons of economics, he offered them alongside premium ready-to-wear clothing.

Over the years, he had built up a growing clientele, hired a seamstress and additional sales staff. The business flourished, time passed and the store began to show signs of wear and tear.

Florian, who had a highly developed sense of aesthetics, was fully aware of this. He had already commissioned two different architects to come up with renovation plans. None of the proposals convinced him. Absorbed in everyday life, he failed to give timely feedback. Embarrassed, he did not get back to either of the architects.

Time passed, gradually the shop began to take on a charmless vintage air. His well-heeled—in both sense of the words—clientele expected a more pleasant ambience with more comfort. Florian was also doubly ashamed, both for the condition of his business premises and for the fact that he had not yet started the renovation.

This was the point at which we discussed the possibilities open to him. As with every ADHDer in this kind of situation, the first step was for Florian to understand how his ADHD functioned. He learned to understand that his procrastination had nothing to do with laziness, lack of character or incompetence. Step by step he got in touch *emotionally* with his own worth, capacity and professional potential.

Having *emotional* access to his own value created a basis for Florian not only to recognise the technical possibilities, but also to overcome his resistance to using them. Without this basis, Florian, like most ADHDers, would have misinterpreted the use of support as questioning his own worth.

The rest of the story is easily explained. We established a living appointment calendar. In this case, not with an external coach, but with one of Florian's employees. At first Florian was concerned that this would undermine his authority—a temporary relapse into his old feelings of self-doubt. However, he quickly managed to adjust his attitude and to focus on the fact that it was an expression of his wittiness to outwit one negative side of his ADHD condition.

One of the shop assistants was brave enough to take on the role of giving Florian the impulses for the renovation work. This naturally took place during working hours and was confirmed to be among her duties in writing. It was agreed that if the project was successful, a special appreciation would be recorded in an interim reference and integrated in her final reference at a later date. This was therefore a classic opportunity for both parties to benefit.

Florian stayed in control of the decisions, but he had to make them by the agreed times. The task of the impulse giver was to remind her boss of the agreed deadlines.

Florian was also prepared to make a supplementary agreement. Should he fail to make and communicate decisions in time, despite everything, then the decision-making authority for the respective step would fall to the respective staff member. This developed into a kind of rivalry, an additional motivational aid.

The success was resounding. The renovation was completed within 7 months.

Yes indeed!

This case study is therefore entitled "The brave tailor", with no talk of a "little tailor" (as in the famous fairy-tale by the Brothers Grimm). Florian faced his no-goes with pragmatism, trusted his potential and proved that he was more courageous than he himself had first suspected.

Just a typical ADHDer.

References

Barkley RA. ADHD through lifecycle—new developments and new trends in diagnosis and treatments. Bern: Workshop Swiss Society for ADHD; 2011.

Biedermann J. Impact of comorbidity in adults with attention-deficit/hyperactivity disorder. J Clin Psychiatry. 2004;65(3):3–7.

Döpfner M. ADHS von der Kindheit bis ins Erwachsenenalter. Psychotherapie im Dialog. 2011;12(3):212–6.

Grolimund F. Vom Aufschieber zum Lernprofi: bessere Noten, weniger Stress, mehr Freizeit. Freiburg im Breisgau: Herder; 2018.

Østergaard SD, Dalsgaard S, Faraone SV, Munk-Olsen T, Laursen TM. Teenage parenthood and birth rates for individuals with and without attention-deficit/hyperactivity disorder: a nationwide cohort study. J Am Acad Child Adolesc Psychiatry. 2017;56(7):578–84.

Philipsen A. Autismus-Spektrum-Störungen und Aufmerksamkeitsdefizit-Hyperaktivitätsstörung. In: Tebartz van Elst l (pub.). Das Asperger-Syndrom im Erwachsenenalter. Berlin: Medizinisch Wissenschaftliche Verlagsgesellschaft; 2013.

Rietzler S, Grolimund F. Clever lernen. Bern: Hogrefe; 2018.

Rist F, Pedersen A, Höcker A, Engberding M. Pathologisches Aufschieben und die Aufmerksamkeitsdefizit-/Hyperaktivitätsstörung. Psychotherapie im Dialog. 2011;12(3):217–20.

Schatz G. Jeff's view: my secret university. FEBS Lett. 2003;540:1–2.

Shaw P, Eckstrand K, Sharp W, Blumenthal J, Lerch JP, Greenstein D, Clasen L, Evans A, Griedd J, Rapoport JL. Attention-deficit/hyperactivity disorder is characterized by a delay in cortical maturation. Proc Natl Acad Sci U S A. 2007;104(49):19649–54.

Sobanski E, Alm B. Aufmerksamkeitsdefizit-/Hyperaktivitätsstörung (ADHS) bei Erwachsenen. Der Nervenarzt. 2004;7:697–716.

Wallis HB, Warner JL, Curtiz M. Casablanca. USA; 1942.

ADHD plays a role in the world of work. Alongside possible everyday disadvantages, the ADHD condition also offers various advantages and great potential. For certain situations, ADHD can even be a decisive success factor. If used correctly, this creates an additional benefit for both the persons affected and the companies employing them.

To follow a successful career path with ADHD, it is important to know how ADHD functions, to know its laws and in particular to understand its cognitive and emotional significance.

It is important to apply this knowledge and understanding not schematically, but always in synergy with the personality and the professional environment of the ADHDer concerned. Communication plays a major role.

This increases the likelihood of better exploiting the person's potential, including in their working life.

In this spirit and by way of conclusion, I propose once again to replace the term attention-**deficit** and hyperactivity **disorder** with the ultimately more appropriate term **Unusual Management of Information and Functions**.

> Attention-**Deficit and** Hyperactivity **Disorder = ADHD**
> or better:
> **Unusual Management of Information and Functions = UMIF**
> *Primary mechanisms (neurobiological)*
> - Information → weighting and filtering:
> - Functions → controlling & dosing
> *Secondary phenomena (reactive and in exchange)*
> - Coping mechanisms
> - Possible side effects of coping mechanisms
> - Misunderstandings
> - Long-term developments and consequences

Index

Printed in the United States
by Baker & Taylor Publisher Services